PAINTING A TARGET ON HPV

Painting a Target on HPV
Published by
Nicholas LeRoy, DC, MS
1002 West Lake St.
Chicago, IL 60607

Library of Congress Control Number: 2015908235
CreateSpace Independent Publishing Platform, North Charleston, SC
ISBN-13: 978-1512231656
ISBN-10: 1512231657

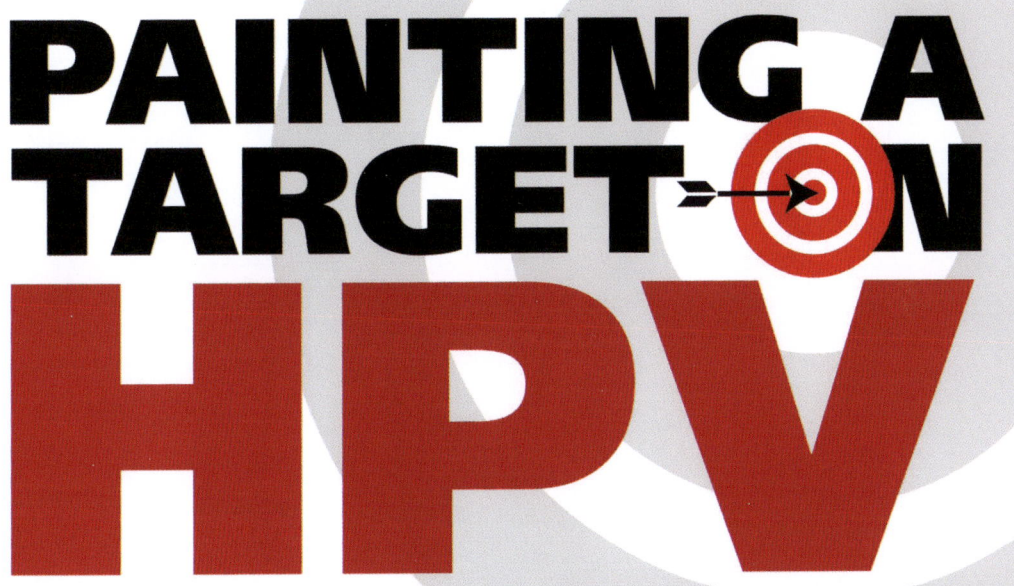

PAINTING A TARGET ON
HPV

Dr. Nick's natural treatment for cervical dysplasia

Nicholas LeRoy, DC, MS
Cover design by Mitch Hagan

DEDICATED TO MY CHILDREN—
Phoebe and Louis

Preface

My journey into the treatment of cervical dysplasia and HPV (human papilloma virus) began in 1995 when asked by a patient if I could help her with mild dysplasia. At the time, I had been in practice for less than a year but had been diligently researching the area of women's health. Why women's health? Simply out of necessity and the drive to help my patients; at that time, the vast majority was women and, in the mid-nineties, there were few physicians who were providing alternative women's health care.

Just months prior to this patient's request for treatment, I had come across literature describing a novel, natural-medicine-based approach for the management of abnormal pap smears. Consisting of two parts, the "indirect" portion utilized dietary and nutritional prescriptions, and the "direct" part consisted of the application of a solution to the cervix that killed abnormal cells. Naturally I was intrigued with this non-surgical alternative.

Armed only with this information—because I didn't learn this treatment in school, nor did I know anyone performing it—I used this therapy successfully and the patient had a normal pap within several months. At the time, I was publishing a monthly newsletter, so I wrote about my success and the treatment; subsequently, *Holistic Chicago* magazine reprinted my article and the rest is, well...history.

It's now about twenty years later and I have successfully treated hundreds of women with cervical dysplasia and HPV. During this time, I have witnessed the suffering of too many women who feel that they have been failed by a medical system reliant on surgical intervention alone. Conventional "wisdom" maintains that there is nothing a person can do to prevent dysplasia or expedite its elimination. I am here to say that this is quite the contrary.

In the nineties, prior to the liquid-based pap test that is now routine, testing for high-risk HPV was not performed, fewer biopsies were conducted, and many gynecologists were treating *all* dysplasia—mild, moderate and severe—with surgery. Since then, our understanding of the condition has changed, resulting in a more conservative approach of "watch and wait", but do nothing, for mild dysplasia endorsed by the American Congress of Obstetricians and Gynecologists (ACOG). In this regard, we have arrived at a more sensible position that performs less surgery and thus, is a good thing; however, the "watch and wait" recommendations often amount to nothing more than to sit on your hands until the condition worsens, necessitating invasive surgery. Additionally, and ironically, this "watch and wait" approach also undermines the success of the future surgical intervention, as those with persistent dysplasia are often more statistically likely to have recurrence after invasive intervention.

This approach is based upon the fact that many women, especially those under the age of thirty, will clear the virus and abnormal cells within a couple of years without any treatment at all. Although on the surface this conservative approach seems wise, it is in fact egregious, as tens of thousands of women each year will not clear the virus and the dysplasia will worsen. When this occurs, a woman's doctor will now insist on surgery, claiming that to do otherwise is reckless, that cancer is going to develop, and that a hysterectomy will be required to prevent death. Well this is quite the change in attitude from that of "don't worry about it, it should go away by itself"!

My position is to treat HPV for what it is: an infection with a virus that is known to cause cancer. As such, treatment to eliminate the virus should begin immediately, not with surgery that does little or nothing to eliminate the virus, but rather to employ dietary changes and supplements to improve immune system function, as well as to treat directly HPV-infected and dysplastic cells. Furthermore, this treatment should be initiated as soon as dysplasia and HPV are identified. This is in direct contradiction to ACOG guidelines that recommend against treatment for mild dysplasia, maintaining the defeatist attitude that everyone gets HPV, that there is no treatment for it, and to not worry about it because it should go away by itself. This is fine, until you are the one in which it doesn't go away and you find yourself ten years and two invasive procedures later, still struggling with recurrent dysplasia.

Conventional treatment ignores the dozens of studies demonstrating that diet and nutrition have a substantial impact on the condition. After twenty years, I have yet to meet with a new patient whose gynecologist recommended something as safe and effective as folic acid, despite the fact that we have known that folic acid deficiency contributes to cervical cancer since the 1960s.

At some point while reading this book you are likely to ask yourself "Why didn't my doctor explain any of this to me?" The answer is straightforward and simple. Conventional treatment and the practice guidelines that dictate treatment recommend no treatment for mild dysplasia and surgical intervention for moderate and severe dysplasia. That's it. In the mind of your doctor, a detailed discussion of HPV and dysplasia is pointless, a waste of his/her time, and isn't going to change how they treat it.

In this book, you will be presented with information to assist you in understanding cervical dysplasia and the virus that causes it. In addition, I will review the comprehensive treatment plan that I have designed, including indirect (oral) and direct treatment modalities for the treatment of HPV-induced cervical dysplasia. Educating yourself will allow you to make treatment decisions based in fact rather than fear. At the end of the day, my goal is to help you to make an informed decision regarding whether you will treat or not treat, and if you do treat, to be confident and comfortable with that decision.

Dr. Nick LeRoy

Contents

Chapter 4
Direct Treatment: Painting a Target on HPV and Dysplasia

Chapter 5
HPV and Cervical Dysplasia Case Studies

Chapter 1-HPV and Cervical Dysplasia: An Introduction

In my twenty years of treating HPV (Human Papilloma Virus) and cervical dysplasia, it has been more than once that a patient has been in my exam room, in tears, confused and scared after being told that she has dysplasia or HPV. The origin of much of this fear and confusion falls squarely on the shoulders of gynecologists; I have found that few physicians take the time necessary to adequately explain this condition, and worse, often give misinformation or bad advice regarding treatment options. Even when pressured by patients for information regarding natural and preventive treatment, doctors nearly always claim that "There is nothing else to do." I am here to tell you that they are completely wrong. You will learn in this book that there are, in fact, many evidence-based strategies that support early treatment with diet, nutrition and other natural therapies.

In this chapter, you will find everything that you need to know regarding HPV and dysplasia to enable you to make good screening and treatment decisions. It is necessary to understand the virus, who it infects, when it infects, and how it transforms a normal cell into a cancerous cell to enable you to make smart decisions regarding treatment. A great deal is actually understood about HPV; however, this knowledge has not changed conventional treatment guidelines that rely solely on surgical interventions, while ignoring decades of published research that should mandate the role of diet, nutrition and natural medicine in the effective treatment and elimination of HPV.

The information provided in this book will enable you to take a proactive role—*to take control*—in making wise decisions in the treatment, elimination, and prevention of HPV and cervical dysplasia. And take control you must, lest you find yourself with recurring dysplasia, while undergoing repetitive surgical procedures that amount to nothing more than a whittling away of your cervix because of bad decisions at the start of it all. Once armed with this knowledge, you will be better equipped to make rational decisions about when and how to treat HPV and dysplasia.

HPV Defined

The Human Papilloma Virus (HPV) is an organism discovered decades ago that is responsible for warts--*all* warts, whether on your feet, genitals, hands or face. HPV is also responsible for a variety of cancers that include the cervix, vagina, vulva, rectum, penis, mouth, throat and lungs. More than 180 types of HPV are known and more are presumed to exist. There are about 40 types of HPV that can infect the anal and genital region with about 14 of them that can lead to cervical, vaginal and vulvar cancer [1].

These potentially cancer-causing viral strains are termed "oncogenic" and can be identified on a liquid pap smear with separate "high-risk HPV" testing. Testing for these high-risk HPVs (HR-HPV) must be requested by the doctor performing the pap but are not typically performed on women under age 30 because there is no medical treatment or prescription drug that is FDA-approved for the treatment of HPV. Women over the age of thirty are more likely to be tested for HPV because an infection is more likely to cause cancer as we age. High-risk HPV strains are more likely to cause cancer, but not warts; and low-risk strains are more likely to cause warts, but not cancer. However, this distinction is not perfect and some low-risk strains may contribute to slowly progressive dysplasia.

It is estimated that up to 80% of the population are current carriers of HPV with active infections that can be transmitted to another person.

Acquiring HPV

A person is usually exposed to HPV by having sexual intercourse, although many of us are first exposed in utero (HPV has been found in amniotic fluid) or at birth when passing through the cervix and vagina. In fact, 30% of children at 2-years of age have evidence of HPV on their genitals and HPV persistence is evident in young girls without any history of sexual activity [2]. HPV can survive on the surfaces of inanimate objects for as long as a week, allowing for potential infection without any direct human contact. If you've walked barefoot in public areas such as showers, you've been exposed to HPV. Sharing of sex toys can expose a person to HPV. Open-mouthed kissing may also result in exposure. And contrary to popular belief, condoms do not prevent HPV transmission because there is still skin-to-skin contact, although condoms may help to minimize exposure to high-risk strains that are more likely to be in high concentration in semen. If you have had sex, it is likely that you've been exposed to one or more strains (it is possible to be infected with numerous strains of both low-risk varieties (warts) and high-risk varieties (cancer). To make matters worse, a person can *auto-inoculate*, transferring the virus from one part of the body, like the vulva, to another part such as the face. This would usually be accomplished by touch.

 If you are freaking out at this point, relax; as you will learn, being exposed to HPV doesn't necessarily result in an infection, an HPV infection will not always cause dysplasia (pre-cancer), and dysplasia will not necessarily result in cervical cancer. The virus is necessary for cancer to develop, but not sufficient, meaning that there are several factors which much coexist to contribute to the infection. There are, in fact, numerous predisposing "co-factors" required for HPV to ultimately cause cancer. Eliminating these HPV co-factors are necessary to treat dysplasia effectively and eliminate the virus from your body. It is my purpose to guide you in this process.

It is important to understand that it can take many years for an HPV infection to become cancerous. Even in cases of severe dysplasia (CIN3), the rate at which invasive cancer will occur if no treatment is performed is estimated to be 12 percent [3]. In other words, there is almost **always** time to undergo natural treatment, even for women with severe dysplasia. The fear tactics employed by conventional doctors to convince women that they will get cancer without immediate surgery, whether intentional or unintentional, lacks scientific credibility. I must point out, however, that the longer you've had dysplasia and the more reoccurrences that you've had, the greater the chance that cancer will develop. Therefore, there is a strong argument to perform a colposcopy and biopsy in women who have a prolonged history of dysplasia (i.e. greater than three years); and perhaps a stronger argument to treat HPV and cervical dysplasia properly at the onset!

In order for the virus to successfully infect the cells of the cervix, it must have access to the deepest layer of the surface tissue or epithelium. This layer, known as the basement membrane, sits beneath the immature stem cells that will mature as they move toward the surface. It is these deep immature cells that are infected with the virus--not the mature surface cells. Thus, it has been postulated that microabrasions of the cervical surface create access to these deeper, immature cells [4]. If cervical micro-trauma is necessary for HPV infection, what is the consequence of grossly traumatic biopsies and LEEPs (Loop Electrosurgical Excisional Procedure)--medical procedures that cut deeply into the cervix?   Is it possible that the medical standard-of-care in evaluating and treating cervical dysplasia is creating more harm than good for some women? It seems likely that medical procedures that cut into the cervix may be contributing to chronic HPV infections and recurrent dysplasia.

Immunity and HPV Infection

The purpose of your immune system is to suppress and kill bacteria, viruses and parasites that find their way into your body. Without a healthy, robust immune system you will die very quickly due to one of the many organisms to which you are exposed on a daily basis, and no amount of antibiotics or antiviral medications will prevent it. This is because even the strongest medications only weaken infectious agents—it's still the responsibility of your immune system to finish the organism off.

There are three basic properties that allow HPV to evade detection and destruction by your immune system:

1. Immune cells circulating in the bloodstream cannot access the virus easily since the HPV doesn't enter the bloodstream. The initial infection is, as discussed, at the basement membrane where there are very few immune cells. Once the virus enters a cell, it is inaccessible to immune cells that cannot give chase. The virus essentially "hides out" and avoids detection by circulating immune cells.

2. As opposed to many other viruses, HPV does not cause major damage to infected cells. If the virus elicited more damage, such as completely bursting open the infected cell, inflammation would result along with an associated increase in immune cells to the site of inflammation. This is what typically happens when the body is invaded by foreign organisms such as cold and flu viruses. However, in the case of HPV, the virus replicates "silently" all the while avoiding detection by the immune system.

11

3. The third mechanism by which HPV avoids immune destruction is via the carefully timed production of viral gene products such as capsid proteins (the outer wall of the complete virus) that are more likely to cause immune detection and subsequent destruction. Rather than produce these capsid proteins early on, they are produced much later in the mature cells of the surface of the cervix to decrease the likelihood of being recognized by immune cells.

If you are wondering why I am discussing what seems to be abstract, there is a purpose to this discussion: If HPV is skilled at avoiding immune system detection and destruction, is there a way to assist your immune system in becoming a better hunter? The answer is yes and methods to improve immunity and bring out the "big guns" will be discussed in detail in chapters 3 and 4. But before we move on to treatment, there is yet more to learn about HPV and how it manages to evade destruction.

Adaptive Immunity Versus HPV

"Adaptive Immunity" refers to the response of the immune system against a specific invader—in this case HPV. It consists of "B cells and T cells". B cells, known also as B lymphocytes, produce antibodies that allow for a highly coordinated attack against a specific organism—sort of like a key fitting only one lock; while T cells, or T lymphocytes, are responsible for "cell-mediated" immunity that is non-specific. Examples of T cells are T-helper cells, natural killer cells, and cytotoxic T cells. It is cell-mediated immunity upon which we are going to focus with regard to treatment because research is finding that T-helper cells are the immune response needed for an HPV infection to be cleared [5]. However, as the reader is likely to suspect at this point, HPV causes a reduction in cell-mediated immunity at the site of an infection.

Cell-mediated immunity plays a pivotal role in clearing HPV. This fact is supported by the observation that HIV- positive persons or those who are immune-compromised due to organ transplant rejection medications, suffer from persistent HPV infections and higher risk of cervical cancer. It is known that AIDS causes a destruction of T-helper cells and an overall decrease in cell-mediated immunity. This decrease is the defining characteristic of AIDS and ultimately results in the death of the individual from a variety of possible infections and/or cancers. The fact that HIV-positive persons have difficulty clearing cervical HPV infections means that the cell-mediated immune activity of the cervix itself is likewise diminished. I point this out because it prompts the following questions: What about HPV-positive, immune-competent persons? Is a less-than-optimal immune system responsible for persistent HPV infections and cervical dysplasia in seemingly healthy individuals? The answer is yes.

Because you are reading this, it is very likely that at some point you were told that you have an abnormal pap. It is also very likely that you were initially told not to worry about HPV and that it should go away by itself. Although it is true that most infections will clear within a couple of years, it is most certainly not due to chance alone. Research has shown that women with HPV16 infections who clear the virus spontaneously have T-helper cells, specific to HPV16, at much higher levels than in women who have persistent infections and severe dysplasia [6]. In other words, women who eliminate the virus and dysplasia without any treatment are doing so because they have a robust immune response. Women who don't clear the virus have a very weak immune response. Therefore, your immune response is an important factor in your ability to eliminate HPV.

Cervical Dysplasia Defined

Cervical dysplasia is a precancerous condition of the uterine cervix caused by HPV. It is identified by looking microscopically at the cells obtained during a pap smear or during a biopsy. An abbreviation for papanicolaou smear, a pap test consists of using a small brush or spatula to scrape off cells from the cervix that are put into a preservative-containing liquid vial (i.e. ThinPrep). This vial is sent to a laboratory where the cells can be placed on a glass slide and screened with a microscope for abnormal cells. A pap test is frequently performed as part of an annual examination that may include a breast exam and a bi-manual examination in which the doctor can palpate your ovaries and uterus. The ultimate goal of performing a pap on a regular basis is not so much to identify cancer, but rather to find *pre*-cancer (dysplasia). Dysplasia means, simply, that the cells are starting to look a bit like abnormal cells but are not quite to the point of becoming cancerous. Cervical dysplasia is easy to treat with early intervention, thereby preventing cancer from ever developing.

The only concern with having dysplasia is that without treatment, some women will develop cervical cancer if given enough time and with the right conditions, such as with nutrient deficiencies, genetic mutations and poor diet.

The initial clue that you may have dysplasia is when you receive an abnormal pap smear result. Although the pap cannot definitively indicate that you have dysplasia, it can show abnormalities suggestive of dysplasia. There are several possible results of a pap smear:

1. **"Negative for intraepithelial lesion":** this means the pap is normal and there are not any abnormal cells visualized with a microscope.

2. **"ASCUS"** (atypical squamous cells of undetermined significance): this finding represents the identification of abnormal cells that cannot be fully characterized. In this event, a colposcopy (staining of the cervix with acetic acid, looking at it with magnification, and likely performing a biopsy) is sometimes performed to better characterize the abnormality. If however, you test HPV negative, the colposcopy may be foregone. ASCUS is a bit tricky to decide follow-up because imbalances in bacteria as well as inflammation can result in ASCUS.

3. " **LSIL**" (low-grade squamous intraepithelial lesion): this pap finding typically correlates with mild dysplasia (remember, think mild *pre-cancer*). The likelihood of LSIL becoming cancer in two years with no treatment is 0.25% [3].

4. " **HSIL**" (high-grade squamous intraepithelial lesion): this finding is suggestive of moderate and severe dysplasia but cervical cancer cannot be ruled out except with a colposcopic biopsy. The likelihood of HSIL becoming cancer in two years with no treatment is 1.4% [3].

The above terminology refers only to squamous cells—the majority of cells found on the outer cervix; however, there is another cell type in which abnormalities can occur, albeit much less often: *glandular* cells. On a pap, glandular abnormalities are described as **AGC** (atypical glandular cells) and **AIS** (adenocarcinoma in situ). AIS is cancer of the cervix that has not spread into the deeper part of the uterus.

It is common to screen for high-risk HPV strains at the time of the pap smear because testing is performed on the same liquid sample. There are thirteen strains of high-risk HPV for which we currently test (16, 18, 21, 33, 35, 39, 45, 51, 52, 56, 58, 59, 68). Strains 16 and 18 are responsible for about 70% of cervical cancer and can be tested for individually, but at the end of the day any of the thirteen strains can cause cancer. We don't test for the forty to fifty low-risk strains that commonly cause warts because their specific identification serves no purpose in the management of dysplasia.

When you receive an abnormal pap it is common to perform a *colposcopic* examination, especially if you test positive for a high-risk strain. The purpose of colposcopy is to apply acetic acid to the cervix, then look at the cervix with magnification. Acetic acid modifies abnormal cells in such a way as to make them appear white, enabling the doctor performing the colposcopy to see areas of dysplasia. It is from the stained areas that a small piece of tissue can be removed and sent to a lab for analysis. Tissue removal and microscopic analysis is known as a *biopsy*, the only way to definitively identify dysplasia and denote its severity. Mind you, however, that the grading of dysplasia from a tissue sample is *subjective,* because it is a *person* visualizing cells with a microscope who then decides what is there. Like most things, there is never 100% agreement from one pathologist to another. Although there are guidelines to maintain consistency in the interpretation and reporting of cervical abnormalities, it remains an educated opinion; there is never perfect agreement between examiners.

The severity of cervical dysplasia, or how close cells are to actually being cancer, is reported in terms of Cervical Intraepithelial Neoplasia (CIN). CIN is a term used in describing biopsy results, not pap results. The severity of CIN is determined by the extent of cancer-like changes on the inside of the cells when visualized with a microscope. Intracellular structures include the nucleus and organelles that perform various functions necessary for the cell to live and to contribute to the sustainability of your entire body. When HPV is driving a cell toward cancer, it causes changes to the nucleus and organelles. One of the key features of dysplasia is an abnormal nuclear to cytoplasmic ratio, or the size of the nucleus as compared to the rest of the cell's interior or cytoplasm. Increased ratios are associated with a greater severity of dysplasia. In addition to the characterization of intracellular abnormalities, CIN grading also takes into account the *thickness* of the lesion. There is a maturation that occurs as deeper immature cells move toward the surface of the cervix, so it is only the deeper cells that should appear immature or undifferentiated. Immature cells near the surface are representative of dysplasia. The scale for CIN is as follows:

1. **CIN1** (mild dysplasia): There is good maturation with minimal nuclear abnormalities. Undifferentiated (immature) cells are confined to the deepest layers. If CIN1 is never treated, there is an 11% chance that it will progress to CIN3 and there is a 1% chance that it will become cancer [3].

2. **CIN2** (moderate dysplasia): Undifferentiated cells extend up to the middle layers of epithelium and there are more marked nuclear abnormalities. If CIN2 is never treated, there is a 22% chance that it will worsen to become CIN3 and there is a 1.5% chance that it will become cancer [3].

3. **CIN3** (severe dysplasia): The entire thickness of the epithelium consists of immature, undifferentiated cells with prominent nuclear abnormalities. If CIN3 is never treated, there is a 12% chance that it will become cancer [3].

4. **CIS** (carcinoma in situ): Cancer that is localized to the surface of the cervix is termed carcinoma in situ (in situ is Latin for "on site"). CIS, by definition, has not invaded into the deeper parts of the uterus. Cancer of the cervix can occur in two different cell types: squamous cells, found on the outer part of the cervix known as the ectocervix; and glandular cells found mainly in the endocervical canal. The former is termed *squamous cell carcinoma in situ* and the latter *adenocarcinoma in situ* (AIS).

5. **Invasive Carcinoma:** This term refers to cancer that is no longer in situ, but has spread beyond the basement membrane and into the tissue of the uterus. If left untreated, it can spread beyond the uterus into other parts of the body that will not be compatible with life (e.g. brain cancer).

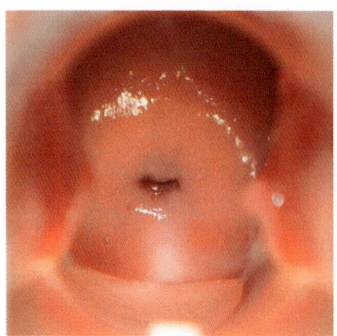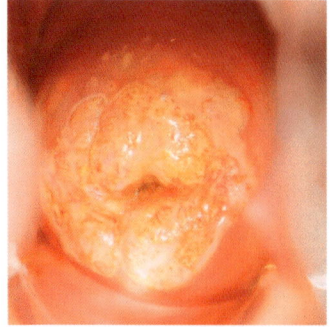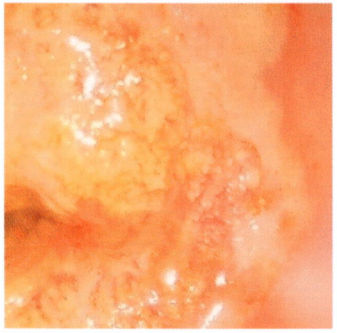

The appearance of dysplasia: The image on the left is the healthy cervix of a 26-year old woman. The center image is the cervix of a 20-year old after the initial application of an escharotic solution containing bloodroot and zinc chloride. Her pap showed ASCUS and a biopsy confirmed CIN1. The areas which appear white are those with HPV-induced dysplasia. The image on the right is a magnification of the right part of her cervix demonstrating *mosaic patterns*, small taste-bud-like projections that are a hallmark of dysplasia.

The Dysplasia Continuum

It is very important to understand that you do not get cervical cancer overnight. Not only does the development of dysplasia (as well cancer) require specific conditions, but it also needs *time*. Cancer never develops from a normal cell without going thru multiple, but seamless, intermediate steps. In effect, there is a continuum of progressively more abnormal cell characteristics that may end in cancer. As discussed above in the "HPV and Cervical Dysplasia Testing" section, the point of a pap is to identify these changes early on so that treatment can be rendered, thereby preventing the development of cancer. This continuum of progressively worsening dysplasia has normal cells on one end and cancer on the other. In other words, cervical cancer is always the result of a gradual progression that starts with HPV infection, then mild dysplasia, moderate dysplasia, severe dysplasia, and finally cancer.

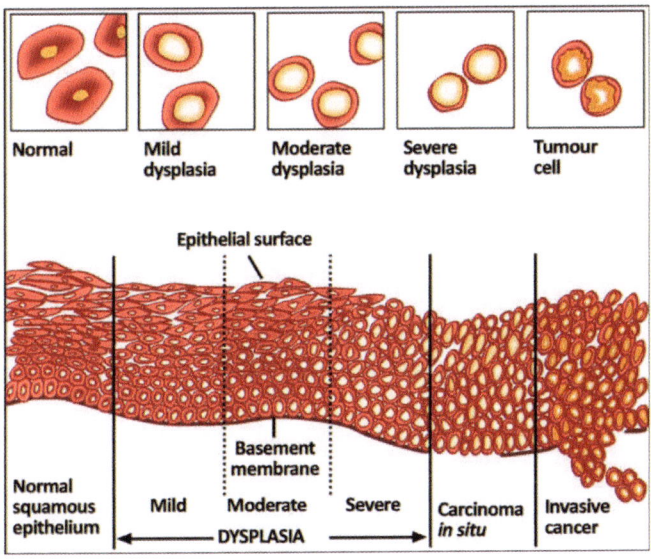

The diagram to the left depicts the surface of the cervix and the progression from a normal cell at the left to cancer at the right. These HPV-induced changes include an enlarging of the nucleus of the cells as well as an increase in the thickness of the dysplastic lesion. This process of ***malignant transformation*** will result in invasive cancer if the process is left unchecked.

Cervical Cancer Defined

Every cell in the human body has a set of instructions within it that determines its function. This "instruction manual" is termed the *genome* and consists of all of the thousands of genes that give us our physical characteristics. Thus, each cell contains within it the entire human genome and the function of any given cell is determined by which genes are turned on and off. Some of these genes are responsible for telling the cell when to grow and when to die and are termed *tumor suppression genes*. Almost all cells eventually die and are replaced by new cells—a process that is controlled largely by tumor suppression genes. They are so important in protecting you from cancer that researchers have dubbed them "guardian angel genes".

Cancer occurs when tumor suppression genes are damaged or inhibited resulting in unchecked cell growth; the cell cannot die and continues to replicate itself eventually forming a mass of malignant cells. In addition to unregulated growth, cancer is best-defined by its lack of respect for anatomic boundaries, possessing the ability to "eat" thru bodily structures spreading to other parts of the body. This last characteristic, known as *metastasis,* is what makes cancer deadly: it spreads into other organs destroying tissue and impairing function which ends up being incompatible with life. Cervical cancer is no different. However, unlike most other cancers, cervical cancer begins with a viral infection—more specifically, a human papilloma infection (HPV). HPV has the ability to *transform* a normal cell into a cancerous or malignant cell.

From Bad to Worse: Malignant Transformation

Being infected with HPV seems bad, but HPV is completely and utterly of no concern—if it weren't for the fact that it has the ability to cause cancer. Cervical dysplasia is also of no concern—if it weren't for the fact that dysplasia represents cellular abnormalities that are moving toward cancer. My point is that HPV and dysplasia are not the problem; the problem is the continued modification of the growth-regulating machinery inside of cells that will ultimately create a malignancy. **HPV literally transforms a normal cell into a cancerous one.** This transformative process is known as *malignant transformation.* The goal of my treatment is to halt this transformation; but to treat it first requires detailed knowledge of what it is. There are numerous changes that occur within a cell undergoing malignant transformation, some of which are well-understood and some of which are not so well-understood, so I am going to focus on several of the most significant and best-researched mechanisms of how cervical cancer develops. These are the inhibition of tumor suppression genes by viral oncoproteins, oxidative stress and vascular endothelial growth factor (VEGF).

Note to the reader: I will be giving considerable detail regarding cell physiology and cell genetics. My purpose isn't to teach you these subjects but rather to give you enough information to help you to appreciate the rationale and intelligence of natural therapy. In other words, I am attempting to impart to you a conceptual understanding that addresses the frequently-asked-patient-questions: "how does natural treatment work?", and "why don't more doctors recommend this therapy?" Well, here it is...

Malignant Transformation: The Role of Viral Oncoproteins

As previously discussed, there are dozens of Human Papilloma Viruses that can infect us, but there is a fundamental difference between those viruses that tend to cause cancer and those that do not. The high-risk viruses have increased expression of *oncogenes.* "Onco" is ancient Greek for cancer, so literally we are talking about viral cancer genes. Just as we have genes to *protect* us from cancer, HPV has genes that *cause* cancer.

It is known that there are only eight genes that make up the HPV genome (compare that to about 30,000 genes in the human!). The purpose of six of them is to take control of your cell's protein-making apparatus to assemble new viral offspring, as well as make certain that these newly-made offspring can leave your cell without destroying it (this last fact was detailed previously because the failure of the cervical cells to die is one of the reasons your immune system has a hard time recognizing the HPV infection). The last two genes, known as E6 and E7, are the oncogenes to which I have referred. These two oncogenes produce *oncoproteins* (cancer proteins) that disable two important tumor suppression genes: the E6 oncoprotein disables the tumor suppression gene p53; and the E7 oncoprotein disables the pRb tumor suppression gene. Cancer cannot occur without shutting down these genes. So essentially, HPV has the ability to shut off the "safety valves" of the cell which only exist to insure that the cells do not become cancerous.

To summarize, high-risk HPV possesses genes that allow it to take control of the cell that it infects. HPV does this so that it can survive, but in doing this, it damages the genes that you have that prevent cancer. This is part of the overall damage that HPV inflicts on infected cells that may ultimately result in cancer. My reason for having described this in detail (as well as what follows) is because there are dietary and nutritional supplements that are proven to protect these genes and stop HPV from causing cancer. This needs repeating: **there are supplements and dietary chemicals that are proven to prevent cervical cancer by protecting tumor suppression genes.** This research-based, natural medicine treatment for HPV will be discussed in Chapter 3.

Malignant Transformation: The Role of Oxidative Stress

Oxidative Stress (OS) refers to the imbalance between the body's production of *free radicals* and the body's ability to detoxify these compounds or at least repair the damage caused by them. The term oxidative stress comes from the word "oxidation", which refers to the passing of an electron from one thing to another. An example of oxidation is when metal rusts. The rust forms because oxygen steals an electron from iron. In your body, when oxygen accepts an electron it becomes a free radical; so you can think of oxidative stress and free radicals as the potential to "rust" the inside of your body. Free radical sources include those that are externally-derived as well as those that are internally-derived.

External sources of free radicals that increase oxidative stress include drugs, chemicals, pollutants, x-rays and ultraviolet radiation. Internal sources include free radicals created by immune system function, inflammation and energy production. Strange as it may seem, the largest source of free radicals is from breathing. With every breath we take, inhaled oxygen passes through the lungs and attaches to hemoglobin inside of red blood cells where it is carried to every cell of the body. Once inside of the cell, oxygen is the final electron acceptor in the production of energy via the oxidation of glucose. No oxygen--no energy production. The problem is that upon accepting an electron, oxygen becomes highly unstable; it becomes a free radical itself. There are a variety of oxygen free radicals and taken as a group are known as Reactive Oxygen Species (ROS). Often the terms oxidative stress, free radicals and reactive oxygen species will be used interchangeably.

Fortunate for us is the fact that we possess an elaborate antioxidant system that is adequate in dealing with all of these reactive species. Adequate, but not perfect, or else we would not age (aging is largely a product of oxidative damage). An example of an intracellular antioxidant is *manganese superoxide dismutase* (MnSOD), a powerful ROS scavenger. You will discover in Chapter 2 that a mutation in the gene that makes MnSOD, when combined with low levels of dietary antioxidants, contributes to CIN and cervical cancer.

Whether derived from outside of the body or generated internally as part of normal bodily function, free radicals damage just about everything with which they come into contact. This includes cell membranes, proteins, mitochondria (the energy making factories of the cell) and DNA. Free radical damage to DNA is perhaps the most alarming consequence of oxidative stress because of the potential for gene mutations that result in cell immortalization (cancer).

If you hadn't already guessed it, HPV increases oxidative stress within infected cells. A 2014 study published in the Journal of Virology found that the HPV E6 oncogene was responsible for decreasing the production of superoxide dismutase and glutathione—two important ROS-scavenging antioxidants—that resulted in increased oxidative stress and DNA damage. The same study also found that this increase in oxidative damage facilitated HPV DNA integration into the host cell [7]. In other words, higher amounts of oxidative stress make it more likely that a person will have a persistent HPV infection with an increased likelihood of developing severe dysplasia and cervical cancer. To further add insult to injury, the E6 oncoprotein diminishes the ability of the infected cell to repair DNA damage, resulting in facilitated malignant transformation [8].

The HPV E7 oncoprotein has also been shown to participate in an increase in aerobic glycolysis within cervical cancer cells [9]. Almost all of the energy produced within our bodies is accomplished aerobically, or with oxygen. When oxygen is limited, such as with intense anaerobic exercise, we switch to glycolysis, which is an inefficient means to obtain energy but does not require oxygen. A by-product of glycolysis is lactic acid—the main reason why we get muscle soreness after intense exercise. A fundamental characteristic of cancer is the fact that there is an increase in glycolysis *despite* adequate levels of oxygen. This phenomenon of glycolysis despite sufficient oxygen occurs in all tumors and is known as the *Warburg Effect*. The Warburg Effect explains the observation that cancer creates an acidic environment within a tumor and surrounding tissue. A physical interaction has been shown to occur between the E7 oncoprotein and enzymes that favor glycolysis over aerobic energy production. **In other words, HPV participates directly in sustaining cancer via the Warburg Effect.**

Note to the reader: Otto Warburg won a Nobel Prize in 1931 for his work on aerobic glycolysis and cancer; however, his findings are often misinterpreted or misrepresented as to mean that cancer grows in an acidic environment. Wannabe advocates of alternative medicine who troll the internet for information that they are not capable of understanding are often keen on exclaiming that cancer grows in an acidic environment, further making nonsensical claims that cancer cannot grow in an alkaline environment. The fact is that cancer doesn't grow in an acidic environment, it creates an acidic environment; and furthermore, to claim that cancer cannot grow in an alkaline environment is ridiculous because you cannot grow in an alkaline environment. Your body has numerous mechanisms to regulate pH—keeping it at 7.4. Any significant departure in pH from 7.4 will result in coma and death.

Malignant Transformation: The Role of VEGF (Cancer Needs Blood to Grow)

As discussed previously, one defining characteristic of cancer is rapid, uncontrolled growth; but to sustain such growth requires additional energy. Because energy that is obtained from the food that we eat is transported to every cell in the body via blood, it stands to reason that an increase in blood flow must accompany the development of cancer. This increase in the flow of blood is accomplished with the growth of blood vessels and is termed *neovascularization*. Neovascularization literally means "new vessel formation", and it is accomplished with *Vascular Endothelial Growth Factor.*

Vascular Endothelial Growth Factor (VEGF) is one of a few chemicals that are produced in cancer cells that increase blood vessel formation to nascent tumors. HPV oncogenes have been shown to induce VEGF production in cervical cells early in the process of malignant transformation [10]. In other words, the production of VEGF occurs soon after infection with high-risk HPV and continues to increase as the dysplasia worsens.

Conclusion

The prospect that the cells of your reproductive system are mutating into cancer by an unseen virus is very frightening. Know, however, that HPV can be stopped. The purpose of Chapter 1 was to ensure that you have enough background information about HPV, dysplasia and how HPV causes cancer so that you may understand the rest of this book, how natural treatment works and why the natural treatment for HPV and dysplasia should be the standard-of-care in treatment. **You will find in the remaining chapters of this book that you are in control of your health and that the means to reverse dysplasia and eliminate HPV is yours for the taking.** The sooner that you become proactive--in contradiction to what you were likely told by your doctor--the sooner that you will eliminate HPV and dysplasia, as well maintain bodily conditions that will prevent its return.

Chapter 2-HPV Cofactors and Predisposing Factors: Partners in Crime

I'm going to let you in on a not-so-little secret: you've been lied to about HPV, cervical dysplasia and cervical cancer. The truth has been completely hidden from you. It may be shocking for you to learn that HPV is **not** the cause of cervical dysplasia and cervical cancer as you've been led to believe. No, that was not a typographical error: HPV is **not** the cause of cervical cancer —at least not **by itself**. The vast majority of the time a person will contract HPV and eliminate it within a couple of years without any treatment at all.

However, there are some patients—about 10-20%--in which the virus will persist, dysplasia will develop, and the severity of the dysplasia will worsen. For these unfortunate women, invasive surgery that can scar or mutilate the cervix is always the recommended treatment. And even with this aggressive treatment, many will continue to have persistent HPV infections, recurring or worsening dysplasia, and the insanity of a repetitive cycle of biopsy, followed by LEEP, followed by biopsy, followed by LEEP and so on. I claim that you've been lied to because a lie it is. All gynecologists are aware of what I am going to tell you in this chapter regarding the necessary cofactors for HPV progression; they simply choose, with some exceptions, to not tell you. I am most certainly not saying that medical gynecologists are untrustworthy or malicious, just that they are handcuffed by their standard-of-care and as a result are hesitant to share some information. **In this chapter, I will detail the research that has found many factors that are necessary for persistent HPV infection, the development of dysplasia, as well as a worsening of dysplasia.**

Knowing that most women with a HPV infection will not develop severe dysplasia and that the vast majority of women will never develop cervical cancer begs a fundamental question. **Why is it that some women have a problem with the virus and some do not?** The answer lies with the simple fact that we are all very different. Some of this difference is due to genetic factors and the rest is due to lifestyle factors. With regard to cervical cancer, some of the contributing genetic factors have been discovered, and they will be discussed. Lifestyle factors are numerous and include diet, nutritional deficiencies, smoking, oral contraceptive use and excess body fat. It is fortunate that most of the factors that cooperate with HPV to cause cervical cancer are modifiable, and if addressed soon after infection they will substantially reduce the likelihood of having long term problems.

For the purpose of this discussion I have divided the factors that collaborate with HPV to cause cervical cancer into two groups: cofactors and predisposing factors. I have chosen make this distinction because cofactors, if not absolutely necessary for disease progression, are very close to being necessary; without them the likelihood of developing cancer is slim. Predisposing factors, on the other hand, do not seem to be necessary but research has demonstrated that they certainly make it more likely that HPV will persist, dysplasia will worsen and cancer will result.

HPV Cofactors for Cervical Cancer: Estrogen and Folic Acid Deficiency

Estrogen: The Good, the Bad and the Ugly

Estrogen is a sex steroid hormone found in men and women that has a multitude of functions. In women, estrogen is produced almost exclusively in the ovary and it is the primary hormone that drives sexual maturation by stimulating breast and nipple development, uterine growth, widening of hips, and enlargement of the vulvar labia. Estrogen is also necessary for the proper development of the endometrial lining that occurs on a monthly basis in preparation for pregnancy. So in other words, estrogen is necessary and important for female puberty and the maintenance of everything that is female; however, this hormone that is necessary and good can become bad under certain circumstances. An example of a negative effect of estrogen is with regard to breast cancer, in which the majority of these cancers are stimulated by estrogen. A significant strategy in breast cancer treatment is to substantially reduce estrogen with drugs and/or the removal of the ovaries.

In a similar manner, estrogen is intimately involved with the HPV-driven changes in the cells of the cervix that results in cervical dysplasia as well as cervical cancer. It is a necessary cofactor for malignant transformation and without it there would be little, if any, cervical cancer. **There are now many studies that have identified estrogen as a cofactor and there is both circumstantial and direct evidence that supports this finding.**

The most compelling circumstantial evidence is that the most estrogen-sensitive region of the cervix is the *transformation zone*, the location of greater than 90% of dysplasia and cervical cancer [11]. The transformation zone is the area adjacent to the endocervical canal where there is a transition from one cell type (squamous) on the surface of the cervix to a different cell type (columnar) found in the canal. This zone is also known as the *squamo-columnar junction*. Apropos to this discussion is the fact that estrogen, as it is metabolized or broken down, can be converted into a couple of different estrogen metabolites, one which is good and the other is bad.

The good estrogen metabolite is 2-hydroxyestrone and the bad is 16-alpha-hydroxyestrone. Studies have shown that the ratio of these two metabolites is a significant factor in the development of a variety of cancers that include the breast, cervix and prostate. The point of mentioning this ratio of good to bad estrogen metabolites is two-fold:

1. The transformation zone described above displays a high level of conversion of estrogen to 16-alpha-hydroxyestrone (bad estrogen) and there is a 700%

increase in this activity when HPV-16 infects and immortalizes these cells. In other words, **HPV modifies the cell that it has infected to produce a large quantity of bad estrogen that pushes the cell further toward cancer** (i.e. it facilitates malignant transformation).

2. The ratio of good and bad estrogen metabolites can be modified with diet and supplementation providing a viable treatment strategy.

The HPV-16 transgenic mouse model exemplifies direct evidentiary support of estrogen as a cofactor in the development of cervical cancer. This mouse has been genetically altered to have the genes from HPV-16 that when exposed to estrogen will develop cervical cancer, and continued estrogen exposure will prevent the cancer cells from dying. If all estrogen is removed, however, the mouse will never develop cervical cancer [12]. The use of these genetically modified mice dates back to the 1990s and provides some of the most compelling evidence that estrogen is necessary for HPV malignant transformation of cervical cells.

More recently, details have been discovered regarding the cooperation of estrogen and HPV. As discussed in chapter 1, there are eight genes that make up the virus with two, E6 and E7, classified as oncogenes—genetic coding sequences that are responsible for cancer formation. **It is now known that estrogen is necessary for the E7 oncogene to degrade the pRb tumor suppression gene.** Recall that pRb is one of the *Guardian Angel genes* that regulate cell division, telling the cell whether to live or to die. In the absence of estrogen the E7 oncogene cannot function and malignant transformation is substantially impaired.

Folic Acid Deficiency

Folic acid, or folate as it is also termed, is a B vitamin that has a vast array of functions in the body. Humans are unable to synthesize it so it has to be gotten through diet or with supplementation. Foods that are high in folate include dark green leafy vegetables, fruits, beans, nuts, meats and eggs. Avocado, spinach, liver, yeast, asparagus, and Brussels sprouts are among the foods with the highest level of folate. Folic acid deficiency is associated with a type of anemia, weakness, nerve damage, depression, mental confusion, mouth ulcers, and behavioral disorders. Deficiency can also cause elevated homocysteine, a chemical that damages blood vessels increasing the risk of heart disease and stroke. It was discovered in 1960 that folic acid deficiency was the cause of neural tube defects in developing fetuses and is one of the main reasons that most countries fortify foods with folic acid and give mothers-to-be vitamins containing folate. Important to this discussion is the fact that folic acid deficiency has been correlated with a number of pre-malignancies and malignancies that include cervical dysplasia and cervical cancer.

Folic acid deficiency has been correlated with cervical dysplasia as early as 1966 [13] but it wasn't until recently that the mechanism was understood: This vitamin is extremely important because of its involvement with DNA methylation. Methylation is the process of adding a methyl group—a carbon and 3 hydrogen atoms—to something during a chemical reaction. Methylation occurs in many reactions throughout the body, and alterations of DNA methylation have been recognized as an important component of cancer development [14]. A more elaborate discussion of methylation as it relates to cancer is necessary to fully appreciate the significance of folate, methylation and cancer formation.

Although we inherit one half of a set of genes from each parent, making one whole set, these genes are modifiable--they can be turned on and off. This is actually a very big deal because for many years it was thought that a person was the sum of their genes, an inescapable fact that would mean that if you inherited a "heart disease gene", for example, you were cursed to die of heart disease. Or if you inherited the diabetes trait you would get diabetes. The reality is that it is much more complicated and the discovery of how methylation turns genes on and off has given rise to the field of *epigenetics*, the study of how exposure to nutrients, chemicals, vitamins, stress and hormones can modify our genetic expression (i.e. phenotype) via methylation of various regions of DNA. It turns out that we are the sum of *both* our inherited genes *and* our lifestyle (and your mother's lifestyle while she was pregnant with you!).

As discussed previously, one of the main features of malignant transformation of HPV-infected cells is the destruction of tumor suppression genes such as p53 and pRb. These genes can be "silenced" when HPV oncogenes modify the amount of methylation of the tumor suppression genes. Gene silencing is known to occur in a number of cancers and is likely involved in *all* cancer development [15]. The importance of folic acid and methylation, however, is not limited to malignant transformation. Studies have demonstrated that the amount of folic acid in your body is an important factor in determining whether or not you are infected with HPV upon exposure.

Exposure to HPV does not guarantee infection. It appears that folate and its promotion of methylation of DNA in HPV-exposed cells helps to prevent against infection. HPV infects a cell by inserting its own DNA into the DNA of a healthy cell. Once infected, the cell will now produce the virus unknowingly and the potential arises for malignant transformation. But if there is sufficient methylation of key areas, the insertion of the viral DNA is impaired and HPV infection is made more difficult. This finding merits repeating: **exposure to HPV does not guarantee infection, folate levels are an important factor whether the virus is able to infect you.** Research has found that women who have *higher levels* of circulating folic acid have a lower likelihood of becoming positive for HR-HPV infection, a decreased chance of having a persistent HR-HPV infection, and a greater likelihood of becoming HR-HPV negative [16].

It is evident that folic acid protects against HPV infection and viral persistence, while at the same time increasing the likelihood of eliminating the virus, but the correlation does not end here: *Folic acid deficiency* has also been shown to increase the risk for dysplasia and cervical cancer [17,18,19,20]. In fact, women who have HPV-16 and *low* levels of folic acid are significantly more likely to be diagnosed with CIN2 or greater dysplasia than are women with HPV-16 who have *higher* levels of folic acid [17]. But recent studies are demonstrating that what really matters isn't just *how much* folic acid you have but *how well* it does what it's supposed to do. This is because folic acid requires an enzyme to do its job but about half of the population has a genetic mutation that impairs the enzyme. This mutation, as well as other mutations that affect HPV, are discussed in the following section.

Predisposing Factors

MTHFR Mutations

I've outlined the significance of folate and how it seems to protect cervical cells from HPV infection and cervical dysplasia by increasing methylation in some areas of DNA while decreasing it in others. What I failed to mention is the fact that many of us cannot reap the benefits conferred by folate because of a mutation in the gene that produces an enzyme critical to folate activity and methylation. This enzyme is methylene tetrahydrofolate reductase (MTHFR) and is necessary to convert folate into its "active" form of 5-methyl tetrahydrofolate. In this activated form it is able to provide methyl groups for cervical cell DNA (this actually occurs via several biochemical steps that is outside the scope of this discussion).

About 50% of us have a MTHFR mutation and it puts us at risk for numerous other diseases that include heart disease, stroke, colon cancer, breast cancer, mood and psychiatric disorders, diabetes, osteoporosis and many others. Clearly, the process of methylation is important in human physiology. There are a handful of studies including a literature meta-analysis in 2013 that demonstrated a correlation between the mutation of MTHFR and cervical cancer [21]. Folic acid supplementation and how to bypass the MTHFR mutation will be discussed in Chapter 3.

Other Mutations?

The existence of the MTHFR mutation may help explain why some healthy women who have great diets and take care of themselves will not clear HPV from their bodies and go on to develop severe dysplasia; while there are other women—women who do not have healthy lifestyles, perhaps who smoke and eat junk food—who readily clear the virus without so much as a hiccup of concern. This can be quite frustrating if you are doing everything that is supposed to help while the results for which you are looking are not forthcoming. It is on a daily basis that a new patient describes the litany of supplements, immune system stimulants, and plant-based diets replete with green smoothies and salads—all the while lamenting: "Why is it that I am not getting rid of this? I never get sick, exercise, take care of myself and I have a great diet. I don't understand!" Genetic variability may hold the key; or perhaps more specifically, genetic mutations.

I've already outlined how folic acid levels are important in HPV infection as well as the transformation of an HPV-infected cell into a dysplastic cell. I've also explained how even a very healthy diet with an abundance of folate-containing dark green vegetables may be ineffective if you possess the MTHFR mutation. But if there is one type of mutation that predisposes you to cervical cancer, might there not also be other mutations that likewise put you at risk?

The answer is yes, and the mutations to which I am referring are actually *single nucleotide polymorphisms*, known as SNPs (and pronounced "snips"). Nucleotides are the building blocks of DNA. One nucleotide is always bound to another nucleotide and strung along in a chain that comprises a single gene. No matter what the gene, it codes for a specific protein that will have a specific duty. For example, the MTHFR gene produces a protein that attaches a methyl group to folate, as described previously. If however, there is a SNP in the gene—in other words a single nucleotide was replaced by a different one—the resulting protein that is made from this now faulty gene is different and cannot properly do its job. There are thousands of SNPs that occur in the human genome, some of which are actually good and may protect us from certain diseases. Many however, are bad.

Rather than describe in detail all of the SNPs that relate to cervical cancer, I will give a brief explanation of a few--not because knowledge of them will necessarily change how you treat dysplasia or cancer, but for completeness of the topic as well as to better understand the genetics of host susceptibility. In other words, this helps to explain why one person has a problem with HPV and another does not.

- **T-lymphocyte mutations**: As previously discussed, cell mediated immunity is diminished at the site of HPV infection. T-lymphocytes, also known as T-cells, are responsible for this very important category of immune system function. A 2014 study found a couple of SNPs in T-cell antigens that can affect cervical cancer susceptibility by altering the immune status of an individual [22]. In other words, there are mutations associated with immune cells that predispose a person to cervical cancer. What is noteworthy is that a person having one of these T-cell mutations would not know it; general immune resistance to cold and flu would likely be unaffected.

- **Cytochrome p450 mutations:** Cytochrome p450 enzymes are detoxification proteins that metabolize or breakdown externally- as well as internally-derived toxins. They are found throughout the body but the majority resides in the liver where about 80% of detoxification occurs, and where the P450 enzymes are responsible for the first step in the detoxification of almost all chemicals and toxins. There are numerous families of these enzymes that do many things in our bodies but for the sake of this discussion, I am referring to the cytochrome P450 1A1 enzymes that break down estrogen and tobacco. Because both estrogen and tobacco are known causes of cervical cancer, the activity of this enzyme would seem relevant. Studies have in fact identified a mutation known as the T3801C single nucleotide polymorphism that significantly increases a woman's susceptibility to developing cervical cancer [23]. Therefore, if you are a smoker with this mutation you are more likely to have a problem with HPV; additionally, if you take synthetic oral contraceptives you may be more likely to have a problem.

- **Manganese superoxide dismutase mutation:** Manganese superoxide dismutase (MnSOD), the primary antioxidant enzyme in mitochondria, plays a key role in protecting cells from oxidative stress. The mitochondria are the energy-making factories of all cells and create free radicals as a by-product of energy production. The cumulative effect of these free radicals is known as *oxidative stress* and was discussed in Chapter 1 as one element of malignant transformation. What is interesting about a SNP in MnSOD is that it isn't correlated with cervical cancer by itself; but rather, this mutation contributes to CIN and cervical cancer *in combination* with low levels of beta-carotene, lycopene, zeaxanthin, lutein and vitamin E [24]. Imagine how this one mutation can confound the results of research investigating the role of anti-oxidants and CIN and cervical cancer: research subjects with this mutation would likely benefit from anti-oxidant supplementation while subjects without the mutation would not; when all the subjects are combined there would be a dilution of positive effect that would make it appear as though anti-oxidants are ineffective at preventing cervical cancer. Now multiply this confusion by a hundred and you'll likely get a better representation of the impact that unsuspecting SNPs have on research in general.

- **Glutathione enzyme mutation:** Glutathione is a very important antioxidant that protects our cells from free radical damage caused by toxic chemicals from the environment as well as free radicals that are created within our bodies. **Glutathione S-transferase M1 null polymorphism** is a mutation in the enzyme that is necessary for glutathione to do its job. Research has found that when this mutation occurs in Indian, Chinese and Southeast Asians the risk of developing both mild dysplasia and cervical cancer is increased. Additionally, all ethnicities that possess this mutation and smoke tobacco are also at increased risk [25,26].

These are just a few of possibly dozens of mutations that predispose a person to persistent HPV and malignant transformation. With the exception of the MTHFR mutation, we do not test for these mutations in a clinical setting. However, knowing whether you posses a SNP is not necessary for the successful treatment of HPV and CIN because natural treatment attempts to account for all possible mutations, cofactors and predisposing factors. This is the defining characteristic of holistic medicine in general.

Additional Predisposing Factors

- **Smoking:** Smoking is the number one cause of preventable deaths in the United States causing almost 400,000 deaths per year. According to the American Lung

Society, cigarette smoke contains more than 7,000 chemicals with 69 of them known to cause cancer. These chemicals include benzene, cadmium, arsenic, formaldehyde and lead. Besides the direct exposure to these cancer causing chemicals, the mechanism of how tobacco increases the incidence of chronic illnesses and cancers consists of the depletion of antioxidants as well as increased oxidative stress. Tobacco smoke with all of its chemicals and toxic metals creates an overwhelming free radical burden to every cell of the body and antioxidants are depleted in an effort to limit the oxidative damage created by this burden. Cigarette smoke has been shown to increase levels of oxidative stress in HPV-infected cervical cells [27].

Smoking has long been recognized as a risk factor for the development of cervical dysplasia and cervical cancer. **A July 2014 study found that tobacco exposure increases E6 and E7 HPV oncogene activity, DNA damage, and mutation rates in HPV-16-infected cervical cells [28}.** This relationship was found to be dose dependent; in other words, the more a woman smokes the greater the ability of HPV to transform her cells into a cancerous ones.

In addition to depleting antioxidants, and perhaps even more relevant to the topic of HPV, is the fact that tobacco lowers folic acid levels [29]. As previously discussed, folate is an extremely important component to methylation. Methylation is a major factor determining the likelihood of HPV infection, the duration of HPV infection as well as the ability of HPV to transform a healthy cell into a malignant one.

- **Air Pollutants:** Tobacco smoke is not the only source of inhaled toxic chemicals. Air pollution has been a characteristic of industrialization and modern living with a significant amount of this pollution attributable to motor vehicles. Research published in the June 2014 edition of *Environmental Health* searched for a correlation between cervical dysplasia and traffic-related hazardous air pollutants. The researchers found that women with the highest residential exposure of benzene and diesel particulate matter had an increased prevalence of cervical dysplasia compared to women with the least exposure [30].

- **Multiple Births:** There is a correlation between multiple births and cervical cancer in HPV positive women. A 2002 study in the *Lancet* found that there was a direct association between HPV infection and the number of births; in other words, the greater the number of births, the greater the likelihood of cervical cancer [31]. A more recent study in the *British Journal of Cancer* found that childbirth increases the risk of developing severe dysplasia (CIN3) among women with persistent HPV infection [32]. *Note that the correlation between number of births and dysplasia and/or cervical cancer is only for women with persistent HPV infections.*

- **Number of Sex Partners:** Obviously the greater the number of sex partners a person has the greater the likelihood of being exposed to HPV. More partners also make it more likely that a person will have multiple strains of virus. For example, a woman can have a low-risk strain of HPV that causes genital warts as well as one or more high-risk strains that cause severe dysplasia. It is conceivable that a person could have 10 or more HPV strains. Barrier methods of contraception (condoms) do not protect against HPV infection since there is normally skin-to-skin contact during intercourse and the virus can be found all over the genital area. Oral sex, as well as hand or finger sexual stimulation, can also spread HPV. Open-mouthed kissing has also been shown to spread HPV. Sex toys can spread HPV if shared.

- **Age at First Intercourse:** Having intercourse before the age of 18 is a risk factor for HPV and dysplasia.

- **Having a Baby Before the Age of 16:** Having a baby before the age of 16 makes it more likely that a woman will have persistent dysplasia.

- **Oral Contraceptives:** The correlation between oral contraceptives pills (OCP) and cervical cancer has historically been unclear. A review of literature published in the Lancet in 2007 that included over 50,000 women in 24 separate studies found an increased risk of developing cervical cancer for current users [33]. This risk was attenuated with cessation of oral contraceptive use. However, since 2007 studies have not been in agreement.

A study published in 2014 concluded that "prolonged use of oral contraceptives demonstrated its benefits in *reducing the risk* of CIN" [34]; while another study, also published in 2014, found that long-term (>5 year), current or recent OCP use has been related to about a *doubling of the risk* of cervical cancer [35]. This apparent contradiction can be frustrating if you are trying to do everything that you can to get rid of CIN and prevent it from becoming cancer. Are OCPs correlated with CIN and an increased likelihood of developing cancer or not? The answer can be found by separating the study participants.

When designing a study, it is the goal of the researcher to account for all confounding variables, so that any difference in the study outcome can be directly attributed to the thing being studied. Part of this can be accomplished by randomly assigning study participants into groups to minimize the risk of differences between a study group and the control group. Another way is to exclude factors that may influence the study outcome. For example, if I am attempting to correlate OCP use with cervical cancer, I may want to exclude from the study all women who smoke, since smoking increases the risk of cancer independent of OC use. The problem arises when there are influencing factors of which we may be unaware. In this case, mutations explain what seemed contradictory and unclear.

There are at least three mutations that, if possessed, will increase the odds that OCP use worsens dysplasia and increases the risk of cervical cancer:

✓ The **MDM2 polymorphism** is a mutation that results in the suppression of the p53 pathway. Recall that p53 is a tumor suppression gene that is important in preventing cells from becoming cancerous. A 2014 study found that there is a synergistic effect between the MDM2 mutation and oral contraceptives in causing dysplasia to worsen [36]. Furthermore, the authors suggested that the MDM2 mutation "might be a good marker for assessing the progression of LSIL to HSIL".

✓ The **interleukin-10 gene polymorphism** has been found to increase the susceptibility to progressive cervical lesions in HPV-infected women who use oral contraceptives [37]. Interleukins are chemicals produced by the immune system that act in the defense of an organism against viral infections.

✓ The **cytochrome p450 1A1 polymorphism**, already mentioned under the topic of mutations, diminishes the ability of the liver to eliminate estrogen from the body. The use of OCP in women who have this mutation increases the risk of developing cervical cancer [23].

Do you need to rush to your doctor to run these tests? No. In fact, these tests are not run in a clinical setting, so you would have a difficult, if not impossible time, getting the tests. My reason for elaborating on the subject of oral contraceptives is two-fold: one, it further underscores the fact that the understanding of all health conditions is always changing and what may seem like fact at one moment in time may turn out to be different than initially reckoned; two, these mutations offer an explanation why some women have more difficulty than others. In other words, the "cookie cutter" approach that defines medicine should be tempered by a lens that acknowledges the diversity and individuality of the host.

My advice is that if you have persistent HPV and/or CIN2 or greater dysplasia and you having been using OC, then stop. For you, the oral contraceptives may be your Achilles heel; it may be the one predisposing factor that is perpetuating the problem.

- **IUDs:** An IUD (intrauterine device) is a small, T-shaped object, slightly less than the length of your pinky that is placed inside the uterus to interfere with pregnancy. IUDs come in two types: hormone-secreting and non-hormone secreting. The hormone-secreting (e.g. Mirena™) releases small amounts of synthetic progesterone (progestin), while the non-hormone IUD secretes nothing. Both physically interfere with fertilized egg implantation within the uterus. It is a form of contraception that has been gaining in popularity because it is easy to use (it can be left in for years) and it is viewed as a way to avoid systemic hormones that may be unhealthy (oral contraceptives). Because an IUD is a constant irritant to the opening of the endocervical canal and the canal itself, it would seem reasonable to think that this chronic irritation may increase the likelihood of acquiring HPV and/or contributing to malignant transformation and a worsening of CIN. This is not the case, however.

A pooled analysis of 26 studies published in 2011 found the IUD use might act to protect against cervical cancer [38]. The authors believed that the chronic irritation may induce local cell-mediated immunity, thereby boosting the local immune response of the cervix. Although the authors' conclusions seem reasonable and as a review the study carries more weight than a single study, things are often more complex when critically evaluated.

In Chapter One I outlined several of the HPV-induced mechanisms of malignant transformation; however, it was a primer on the subject and was by no means a comprehensive outline of *all* mechanisms of malignant transformation. Apropos to the discussion at hand is another finding associated with worsening dysplasia: the change in the expression of sex steroid receptors.

One way in which the growth cervical cells are controlled is via sex steroids (estrogen and progesterone). In a healthy cervix, the cells are estrogen receptor-positive and progesterone receptor-negative. However, in cervical pre-cancer and cancer the expression of estrogen receptors decreases and the expression of progesterone receptors increase; and this change is proportionate to the severity of dysplasia [39]. In mild dysplasia there are minimal receptor changes as compared to a healthy cell but these changes are amplified as the dysplasia worsens.

So in other words, the effects of IUDs may vary according to whether a woman has dysplasia or not. In most women, the irritating, immune-stimulating effect of the IUD may reduce the risk of HPV-induced CIN; but in some women in whom the dysplasia worsens, perhaps because of other predisposing factors, the progestin from the IUD that leaches into the local reproductive tissue may now act as a carcinogen because of the increase in progesterone receptors.

My advice: if you have CIN2 or CIN3 and you have a hormone-secreting IUD you may want to remove it; it's just not worth the potential risk that the synthetic progesterone imparts. Anecdotally, I have had numerous patients with a hormone-secreting IUD who were responding slowly to dysplasia treatment who seemed to do better after the IUD was removed.

- **Unhealthy diet:** We hear and read so many conflicting findings regarding the food that we eat that it is easy to get confused and apathetic. Much of this is due our preoccupation with weight loss and the marketing of weight loss products by businesses attempting to capitalize on this multi-million dollar industry. A healthy diet, however, is characterized more by the level of vitamins, minerals and micronutrients than it is the amount of calories and relative proportions of fats, proteins and carbohydrates. **It's the micronutrients that include complex phytochemicals that help to prevent cancer by inhibiting the processes that are involved in malignant transformation.**

Research has shown that there is an inverse association between antioxidant micronutrient concentrations in a woman's blood and the risk of cervical dysplasia—less antioxidants equals more abnormalities. The specific dietary antioxidants that have been correlated are beta carotene, lycopene, zeaxanthin, lutein, vitamin A, and vitamin E [40]. **A study in the *International Journal of Cancer* found a 50% decreased risk of developing CIN3 with a higher dietary intake of dark green and deep yellow vegetables and fruits [41].** Folic acid and B vitamins are found in dark green vegetables while the carotenoids that include beta carotene, lutein, zeaxanthin, vitamin A and lycopene are found in the yellow-orange vegetables. If higher levels of these nutrients obtained from a healthy diet help to prevent severe dysplasia, then it is reasonable to think that diets lower in these nutrients are a predisposing factor for a worsening of dysplasia.

The correlation between an unhealthy diet and CIN risk is more than just preventing oxidative stress by eating a lot of antioxidants; your diet also influences the ability of your body to properly methylate. Recall that methylation of DNA is critical to determining how your cells behave including the proper functioning of tumor suppression genes that prevent cells from growing uncontrollably. Methylation can also prevent HPV infection, and once infected methylation is involved in diminishing the activity of HPV oncogenes. We've discussed previously how the B vitamins--and folic acid especially--are necessary for methylation; but from where are these vitamins normally obtained? Your diet! More specifically, your *healthy* diet. A study published in 2012 looked at the degree of methylation as it relates to diet and CIN and found that women with unhealthy diets, low in fruits and vegetables, had much lower methylation in the body. **Furthermore, these same women with the unhealthiest diets were 3.5 times more likely to be diagnosed with CIN2-3 than women with the healthiest diets and most methylation [42].**

A great deal more of this will be discussed in the following chapter including how a plant-based diet, replete with dark green leafy vegetables and fruits, makes it more likely that you will eliminate HPV.

- **Low or Compromised Immunity:** It is cell-mediated immunity that is necessary to eliminate an HPV infection. In the event that HPV becomes persistent and the process of malignant transformation begins, it is also cell-mediated immunity that is called in to destroy these abnormal cells. As discussed in Chapter 1, HPV has a knack for diminishing cell-mediated activity at the site of infection and this, combined with the fact that the virus also evades detection because the infected cell are not destroyed, leads to viral persistence and dysplasia. All of this occurs even in healthy individuals with competent immune systems; but in women with compromised immunity it is much worse.

  Women with HIV, AIDS and those who are taking medications to suppress immunity have much higher rates of HPV persistence, cervical dysplasia and cervical cancer. Immunosuppressive drugs are used after organ transplant surgery to prevent organ rejection and with autoimmune diseases such as rheumatoid arthritis as well as immunity-related disorders such as psoriasis. HIV causes T-helper cell destruction and the lower the number of these immune cells the greater risk of CIN and cervical cancer. **The correlation with immunity and HPV is quite simple: low immune system function equals persistent HPV and increased odds of developing cancer.**

- **Unhealthy Vaginal Microbiota:** There are trillions of bacteria that reside in the mouth, intestine and vagina. Decades of research have correlated normal human metabolism, physiology and immunity with the sum total of these bacteria, known as the *microbiome*. Some bacterial species are correlated with good health while others are the cause of diseases that include obesity, autoimmune diseases, arthritis, cancer, and gastrointestinal diseases. For each of us, our own personal microbiome modifies our immune system, produce vitamins and other chemicals necessary for proper physiology, and maintain the health and integrity of the cells that line the intestine (i.e. the mucosal surface). In fact, the vast majority of chemicals found in our bloodstreams have bacteria as their origin.

  Try to imagine the significance of 100 trillion bacteria in our guts that share with us about 4 million total genes, and contrast that to the mere 26,000 genes that comprise a human. Suffice it to say that the microbiome is the single most important factor in human health and disease. With this in mind, in 2007 an international consortium of researchers began the *Human Microbiome Project* with the goal of characterizing the composition and diversity of microbial communities on the major mucosal surfaces in the human body. The significance of this data in the current context is that bacteria in the vagina impact HPV infections.

  Known as the vaginal microbiota (VMB), the sum total of all genus and species of bacteria in the vagina are more complex than previously thought. To summarize, it has now been conclusively demonstrated that lactobacilli-dominated VMB are associated with a healthy vaginal microbial environment [43,44,45,46] while a loss of lactobacilli and a bacterial imbalance—specifically an increase in microbial diversity—is associated with bacterial vaginosis (BV) [47]. **Significant to the topic-at-hand is that a BV-like vaginal environment is also associated with HPV infection [48,49,50].** In other words, women who have a chronic BV-like vaginal microbial environment are more likely to have HPV as well as HPV persistence.

Similar research has also correlated oral gingivitis with BV [51], suggesting that **oral health may affect genital HPV infections** via a stream of association: gingivitis is correlated with BV and BV is associated with genital HPV, therefore gingivitis contributes to vaginal and cervical HPV. The take away message? Oral health influences the vaginal microbiota which in turn affects the likelihood of HPV infection and persistence.

The Take Away Message

If you have a recent infection with HPV or have been diagnosed mild dysplasia, the odds are that you will not have a problem with the virus or with worsening dysplasia. However, the likelihood that you will have a problem cannot be determined because physicians are unable to account for all predisposing factors. For example, out of the numerous genetic mutations that increase the likelihood that you will have persistent problems, we test for none. Nor do we assess whether you are having micronutrient deficiencies shown to worsen dysplasia. We don't even test for folic acid deficiency—a cofactor for cervical cancer that was established many decades ago—despite the fact that we can easily test for deficiency as well as the folate-associated MTHFR mutation. My point is not that we should do more comprehensive testing, but rather that we should treat HPV and CIN *rationally.*

Does it seem rational to ignore predisposing factors when treating HPV and CIN? Is the conventional do-nothing approach for HPV infections and mild dysplasia *scientific*? You, the reader, can make that determination yourself. **My recommendation is that if you have a recent infection or mild dysplasia, don't do nothing; treat it as though it is going to become a problem so that you will never have to deal with a phone call from your doctor or nurse who exclaims that you have severe dysplasia and must get a LEEP immediately or you are going to risk getting cancer and a hysterectomy.**

If you have had problems with HPV--in other words, if you have had a persistent or recurrent HPV infection and/or CIN2 or worse dysplasia--then you must address *all* of the factors that relate to HPV. **This is the only rational approach. It's the only scientific approach. This is because for you to have worsening dysplasia *requires* that you have a predisposing cause.** Whether it's due to a mutation, a poor diet, oral contraceptives, smoking or an impaired immune system, HPV needs its partners in crime.

Chapter 3-Oral Treatment: Diet and Supplements

In Chapter One, we examined the factors involved in acquiring HPV, HPV persistence, dysplasia and the development of cervical cancer. As part of that discussion, malignant transformation was characterized as a progression of HPV-induced changes that occur inside of the cell that is becoming increasingly dysplastic; if unchecked, this progression will result in cervical cancer. These cellular changes, driven by HPV in its need to replicate are the destruction of tumor suppression proteins, oxidative stress and the production of vascular endothelial growth factor. Malignant transformation is defined by these changes. In effect, HPV hijacks the cellular machinery responsible for normal cell function, replacing it with new programming whose purpose is aligned only with that of the virus: replication and survival. This programming creates a cell that is unable to stop growing, losing all respect for anatomic boundaries. It creates cancer.

In order for HPV to transform a normal cell into a malignant one it must have *time*. **Clear the virus quickly and it will never cause cancer.** If you end up with a persistent HPV infection, you are likely looking at years of screenings, colposcopies, biopsies and surgical procedures—all the while in constant fear that you will develop cancer; so viral persistence is first and foremost the main concern. In Chapter One, in addition to describing the process of malignant transformation, I discussed the correlation of immunity, viral persistence and dysplasia. Weak immunity results in difficulty clearing the virus, viral persistence and an increased likelihood of developing CIN; therefore, immunity must be addressed as part of a comprehensive approach to HPV treatment.

In Chapter Two, HPV cofactors and predisposing factors were described because acquiring HPV alone is not sufficient to develop cervical cancer. **HPV persistence and malignant transformation is much more likely to occur in individuals with poor health, nutritional deficiencies, unhealthy diets low in fruits and vegetables, smokers, and those with impaired immunity.** Addressing these risk factors is smart treatment; ignoring them is not. And yet that is exactly what your conventional doctor does: assure you that there is nothing that you can do to get rid of HPV and that it will go away by itself; and even when you develop mild dysplasia, that same doctor is still insistent upon a do-nothing-treatment-strategy, still proclaiming that there is no need for worry; then suddenly does a 180 degree turnabout when you develop CIN2 or 3, exclaiming that you are going to get cancer and need immediate surgical intervention. This is insanity.

What I've shared with you in the first two chapters of this book served several purposes. The first was to provide you with detailed information regarding HPV, what it is, what is does, and how it does it. Understanding the process of malignant transformation is necessary if you are to appreciate the logic behind dietary and nutritional supplementation. The second was to demonstrate to you that there is published research supporting the role of natural medicine in eliminating HPV and in treating and preventing CIN and cervical cancer. The significance of this fact is not to be overlooked. Most of us assume that a board certified gynecologist is an authority regarding all things gynecological including HPV. It is this assumption that prevents many women from seeking out alternative care. This assumption is incorrect. **Your doctor's recommendations do not reflect what is known about HPV, ignores a vast compilation of research, and is likely to harm you.**

The "Simplicity" of Conventional Treatment

The conventional medical treatment of HPV and cervical dysplasia varies according to the severity of dysplasia as well as the age of a woman, but at the end of the day is actually quite simple: do nothing or cut out part of your cervix. There's no in-between. If you have an HPV infection the recommendation is to do nothing and you will be told that it will go away by itself. When it doesn't go away and you are diagnosed with mild dysplasia, you are again told to do nothing and reassured that it will go away. **But when it doesn't go away and becomes moderate or severe dysplasia suddenly your doctor does an about-face and you are warned that your very life is in danger—that if you don't immediately have surgery you will probably get cancer.** What the heck happened to "don't worry about it"?! If this scenario is all too familiar to you, you are not alone; there are tens of thousands of women every year who end up with CIN2-3 because of bad advice from their doctors. What happened is that you and all of these other women were blindsided by the medical-standard-of-care.

> **Case Study:** Sharon was a 32-year old woman whose first abnormal pap was in 2001. At that time, her doctor recommended to do no treatment and for the next five years she did regular pap smears, some of which were normal and some abnormal. In 2006, Sharon had an ASCUS pap with high-risk HPV that prompted a colposcopy in which the biopsy was normal. One year later she had another biopsy that demonstrated CIN3 and had a LEEP performed. After another abnormal pap one year later she had her second LEEP in 2008. Her pap was normal for one year then had a couple of paps with mild dysplasia with no treatment until 2012 when she had her third LEEP following an abnormal colpo. I first saw her in November of 2014 after a biopsy the month before identified CIN3 again. Now her doctor recommended a fourth LEEP which she refused and sought out my care.

When I first saw Sharon, I suspected that she had the MTHFR mutation considering the recalcitrance of her dysplasia and the HPV persistence. Testing was performed and she did indeed possess the mutation. Treatment consisted of supplementation with DIM, methyl folate, curcumin, a probiotic, vitamin D, a mushroom blend and a multivitamin. An escharotic solution was applied to her cervix approximately once per week until all visible traces of dysplasia were eliminated (it ended up being seven total treatments). Her follow-up pap was normal and there was no high-risk HPV detected.

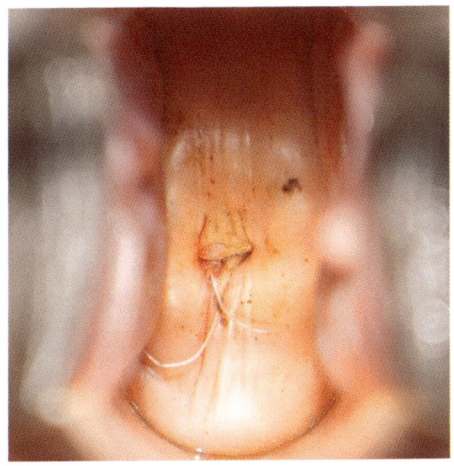 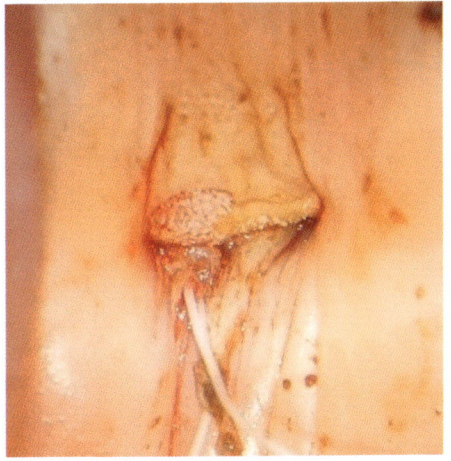

These are the images of Sharon's cervix after applying the first escharotic solution. The area of CIN3 is actually quite small and is limited to the area just above the opening of the cervix. The image on the right is the opening magnified and showing fine *mosaic lesions*—tiny bumps that are the hallmark of dysplasia.

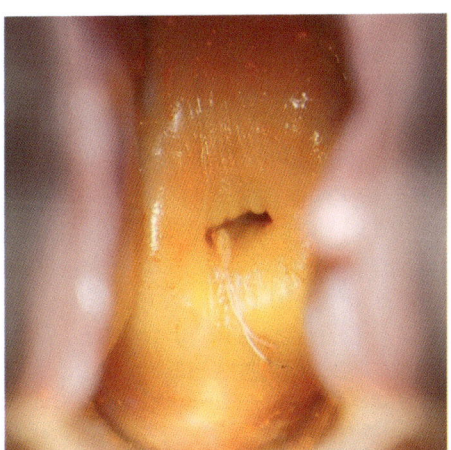 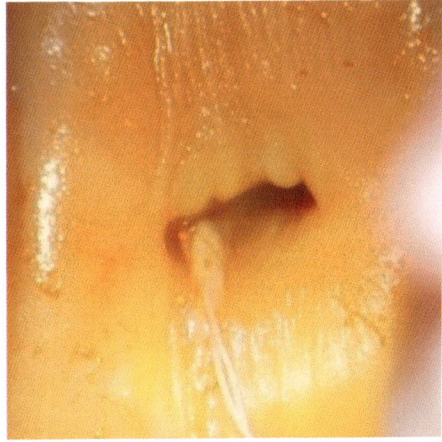

Sharon's cervix appears yellow/orange because of the addition of curcumin to the solution. The image on the right is the same area magnified after four treatments. Note that the lesion is absent. Two more treatment were done because I was suspicious of how quickly she responded and wanted to be certain of resolution before doing a pap (which was normal and HPV negative).

*Sharon's case is a classic mismanagement of HPV and dysplasia. The fact that she had been struggling with this for almost 14 years—having 3 LEEPS, and soon to be 4—is absolutely ridiculous. **When a woman is having persistent HPV there is always a reason; and that reason is not simply bad luck.** Fortunate for Sharon, the doctor who* *did the three LEEPs was not overly aggressive with the amount of tissue removed and her cervix had weathered the abuse fairly well. This is in contrast to other women whom I've seen with similar protracted histories but have been left with almost no cervix or have ended up with hysterectomies.*

Medical Standard-of-Care: The Yoke of Stupid *(at least with regard to HPV!)*

Medical standard-of-care is "a diagnostic and treatment process that a reasonable clinician of that specialty and similar stage of training should follow for a certain type of patient, illness, or clinical circumstance." There are standards-of-care for the diagnosis and treatment of almost all conditions, and they are usually a set of written guidelines that are adopted by the members of a medical specialty that are supposed to reflect the most current understanding of how to diagnose and treat a condition. With regard to the screening and treatment of cervical dysplasia and cervical cancer, **there are two main sets of guidelines that are followed by gynecologists.** One is the American Congress of Obstetricians and Gynecologists (ACOG) and the other is American Society for Colposcopy and Cervical Pathology (ASCCP). These two sets of guidelines are mostly in agreement and literally determine, in detail so specific as to leave almost no flexibility, who should be screened, when they should be screened, what tests should be performed and what is the recommended treatment when an abnormality is identified.

The problem with all standards-of-care is that they are not necessarily supported by research—at least not wholly—but are rather the summation of prevailing thinking by the members of a medical specialty. **This would seem reasonable on the surface, except for the fact that medical specialists, such as gynecologists, are indoctrinated into a medical system heavily influenced by profit and the pharmaceutical industry.** In other words, there can be tremendous bias inherent in standard-of-care guidelines. Don't expect that medical guidelines will include diet, nutrition or anything else holistic and natural.

The inclusion of natural medicine is lacking in all treatment guidelines because there is too little profit in diet and supplements. In fact, a supplement cannot be patented and without a patent, a pharmaceutical company will never recoup their massive investment in getting FDA approval for the treatment of a specific condition. The reason that so many women are injured by gynecologists isn't that gynecologists are bad people, but rather because they must follow standard-of-care or risk medical board sanctions and/or a malpractice lawsuit. **Furthermore, they truly believe that they are doing what is in your best interest, unaware that the guidelines have become a yoke around their necks, stifling creativity and the use of their thinking brains: the Yoke of Stupid.**

Note: *Unfortunately, some women find themselves directly in the crosshairs of doctors who seem to think that their treatment guidelines have been chiseled in stone and carried down from Mount Sinai. The account of one such patient who was "discharged"*

(I say kicked to the curb) by her doctor because she wanted to attempt natural treatment before resorting to a LEEP can be found in Appendix A.

My analysis may seem harsh to the reader but I have little tolerance for those who ignore reality. The reality is, for example, that we've known that folic acid deficiency is associated with cervical cancer for almost fifty years, and yet you were not likely told by your doctor to supplement with folic acid. As discussed in Chapter 2, folic acid deficiency can be considered a co-factor in HPV infection and progression to dysplasia, with decades of research attesting to this fact, and yet you were not told about it. Why not? You've already been given the answer: because the standard-of-care that dictates the treatment of HPV and CIN does not include the use of folic acid nor any other supplements or dietary recommendations. This is not, however, because natural medicine is ineffective in treating HPV; nor is it because there is no proof that they work--because there is a great deal of research attesting to the fact that they do work-- but solely because supplements and diet are not "FDA-approved" for the treatment of HPV and CIN.

The FDA: Consumer Watch Dog?

The Food and Drug Administration (FDA) is a federal agency of the United States Department of Health and Human Services responsible for protecting and promoting public health through the regulation and supervision of tobacco products, dietary supplements, prescription and non-prescription drugs, medical devices, vaccines, food safety and cosmetics. Its primary focus is the enforcement of the Federal Food, Drug, and Cosmetic Act. Dietary supplements including vitamins, minerals, herbs and other plant chemicals are regulated under this act because they are classified as food.

It is an incredibly expensive and lengthy process to discover, develop and launch a drug—estimated by Forbes to cost from $4 Billion to $11 Billion. Much expense is incurred in the early phases of development. For instance, only one out of every ten thousand discovered compounds actually becomes an approved drug for sale, and only 1 out of every 3 approved drugs generates enough money to cover the development costs of previous failures. This means that for a drug company to survive, it must discover a drug that generates billions of dollars in revenue every several years.

You may be scratching your head wondering why I am sharing information about the cost of developing drugs as well as getting FDA-approval when the treatment for HPV and CIN discussed in this book does not consist of the use of prescription drugs. **I am sharing this information because in order for a drug company--or a supplement manufacturer for that matter--to claim that a compound can treat a specific condition such as HPV and CIN, it first must be FDA-approved.** Much of the expense described above is to conduct studies demonstrating the benefit as well as safety of a compound for which a drug company is seeking approval. If a health claim is made in the absence of FDA-approval, the full weight of the FDA will bear down in the form of armed Special Agents of the Office of Criminal Investigations—not something to take lightly.

Without FDA approval, no matter how effective a compound is in treating a condition, it will never be used as treatment because it will never become a part of the standard-of-care. If it's not standard-of-care, your doctor will not recommend it because it will not be included in the treatment guidelines. Sadly, this is the case with much of natural medicine in general. Vitamins, minerals, plant compounds and other naturally occurring chemicals cannot be patented and thus the massive investment in getting FDA-approval cannot be recouped by the patent exclusivity enjoyed by pharmaceutical companies.

*Note to the reader: It's unfortunate that it is so expensive to get FDA approval because there would be a benefit in getting supplements FDA approved. One of the tasks of the FDA is to ensure drug quality and quantity. If a drug says that there is 25mg of the active chemical the FDA verifies this—in other words, there is very good quality control enforced by the FDA. This is not the case for natural supplements, however. In February 2015, the New York States attorney general's office accused four major retailers of selling fraudulent and potentially dangerous supplements, finding that 4 out of 5 of the tested supplements did not contain what was written on the label. The retailers? Walmart, Target, Walgreens and GNC. Now I have to say that if you are buying supplements from these stores what did you expect? Because what do they all have in common? They're CHEAP. Most of us have heard at some time in our lives that "you get what you pay for". There aren't any holistic physicians alive who recommend supplements from these types of retailers. We use products from nutraceutical companies that apply stringent quality control, including chemical assays on all products that are commensurate with that of pharmaceutical companies. My supplements don't cost more than Walmart because I am greedy; they cost more because they are high quality and you can be assured that what is written on the label is in the pill. They tend to be more expensive because they are the real deal.

Much of the remaining part of this book will demonstrate to you the scientific basis for the use of natural substances to treat HPV and cervical dysplasia. **Despite the fact that none of the treatment that I am going to recommend is FDA-approved, that it is not the standard-of-care nor part of the treatment guidelines, that none of it will you ever hear about from your doctor, *it is nonetheless the treatment of choice for HPV and all dysplasia.***

To Treat or Not to Treat?

As previously described, all board certified gynecologists follow the guidelines developed by the American Congress of Obstetricians and Gynecologists (ACOG). ACOG, as well as your doctor acting in accordance with ACOG, would have you believe that to do nothing at all is the sensible approach to HPV and mild dysplasia. I can tell you that after twenty years of caring for women who have been injured by this approach, both emotionally and physically, that it is wrong--wrong and careless.

Although it is correct in acknowledging that most women will eliminate a recent infection with HPV as well as recently-developed mild dysplasia, there are nonetheless millions of women who do not clear the virus and whose CIN1 becomes worse. For these women with persistent HPV and worsening dysplasia, surgery becomes the recommended treatment. "Don't worry, your HPV will go away" becomes "we have to do surgery or you are going to get cancer". I myself, on the other hand, know that prevention is the best medicine. **Early intervention with safe, effective natural treatments for everyone with HPV and early dysplasia eliminates persistent dysplasia and saves thousands of women the fear and pain associated with surgery, HPV recurrence, and further surgery.**

It is important to keep in mind that the Human Papilloma Virus is a cancer-causing organism and should be treated as such. **To recommend no treatment at all for a young woman with a recent HPV infection simply because "everyone has it" is egregious and in some cases portends years of unnecessary suffering, cervical-mutilating LEEPs and conizations, and recurring or worsening dysplasia** (a conization is a more aggressive surgical removal of a cone-shaped piece of cervix that is accomplished with a scalpel or laser knife). Fortunately, the virus can be dealt with, cervical dysplasia can be completely eliminated—all without surgery or drugs—and you can live out your life without looking back over your shoulder. This is the peace-of-mind that I seek to provide to you.

Conventional Treatment of HPV and Dysplasia

Conventional medicine is the prevailing form of healthcare in the West and is rooted in pharmacology and surgery. Historically, it has also been known as "allopathic medicine", a term that means "other than disease", because critics have claimed that the focus of conventional medicine is on symptoms rather than the underlying physiological reasons why a person is sick. Although this claim may have had merit in the 19th century, modern medicine--with the employment of the scientific method--has led to a detailed understanding of human physiology as well as the advancements in the treatment of many diseases. Despite this, and perhaps for this very reason, medicine is reductionist in its methodology. It seeks to reduce a person to his or her illness, often losing sight of the whole person. The fact that the practice of modern medicine is broken into many fields of specialty underscores this trait. If you have a skin disease you see a dermatologist who focuses only on your skin, failing to recognize that the health of your skin is dependent upon your dietary habits and the health of your gastrointestinal system. Similarly, the medical expedient in treating a tumor is to remove it surgically without much thought as to why it developed in the first place. This continues to be the approach to cancer: a slash and burn mentality that disavows the innate capacity of the human body to gravitate toward a state of health (i.e. homeostasis). The conventional approach to HPV and dysplasia is no different.

Most women follow their gynecologist's recommendation and do nothing when first diagnosed with HPV or CIN1. If the dysplasia worsens, your doctor will insist that you have a surgical procedure known as a *LEEP* (loop electrosurgical excision procedure) or *conization* (cone-shaped removal of part of the cervix accomplished with a scalpel). The purpose of either procedure is to cut out the abnormal tissue using an electrified scalpel of sorts. Although most women tolerate a LEEP without too many problems, there is nonetheless potential for infections, scarring and the need to repeat the LEEP because the dysplasia was not fully removed or because the dysplasia comes back. Additionally, having a LEEP may increase the likelihood of having a miscarriage in the future. To add insult to injury, most women are assigned pelvic rest for 4-6 weeks after LEEP surgery— a psychosocial punishment for contracting HPV. Now HPV treatment has made you an invalid for a month or so. In contrast, my natural treatment does not interfere with any of your normal activities.

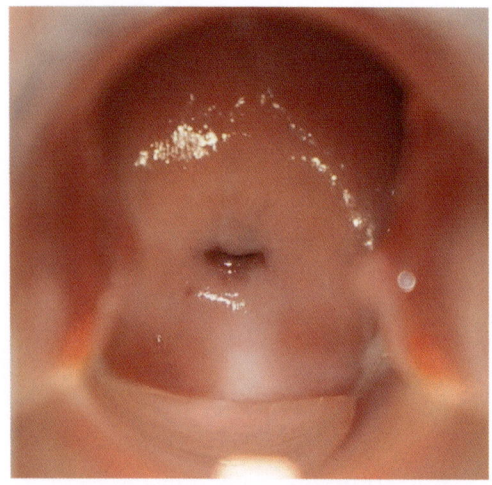

This is the cervix of a healthy 26-year old woman previously treated for CIN2.

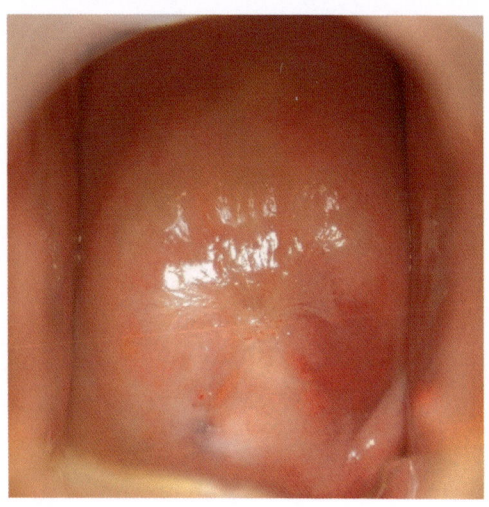

This is the cervix of a 67-year old who had a LEEP for mild dysplasia. Notice something missing? Her endocervical canal closed up after the LEEP, potentially trapping abnormal cells inside of the now inaccessible cervix (there were not "clear margins" on the removed tissue which means that some dysplasia was left behind). So this woman, who really didn't need a LEEP even by medical standards, was faced with the uncertainty of developing cancer inside of the closed cervix. She was considering a hysterectomy in order to not worry about it.

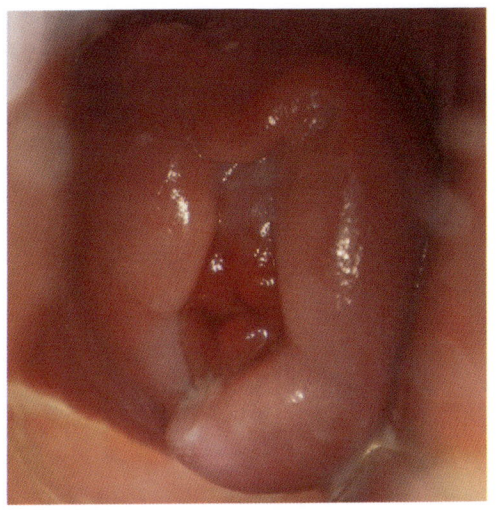

This is the cervix of a 54-year old woman who had a LEEP over 10 years prior. Note the resulting deformity. Although this is not characteristic of most excisional procedures, it does happen.

HPV persistence following a LEEP can be as high as 35% [52]--not a particularly great statistic considering that continued HPV infection makes it more likely that you will develop dysplasia again. In fact, studies have demonstrated that the risk of recurring cervical disease following a LEEP is between 8% and 18% [53,54]. Rates of recurrence are even higher with conization procedures, however.

Conization is the removal of a large, cone-shaped piece of tissue from the cervix. It is another commonly performed surgical treatment for CIN, but is also sometimes used to obtain tissue to examine microscopically as part of a biopsy. It is a more aggressive version of a LEEP and sometimes consists of the entire removal of the ectocervix (the part of the cervix that is visible in the vagina). Rates of recurrence of disease can be as high as 32% following a "cone", as it is sometime termed [55]. High recurrence rates of dysplasia following LEEPs and cones, as well as HPV persistence, question the wisdom of the medical management of HPV-related cervical disease.

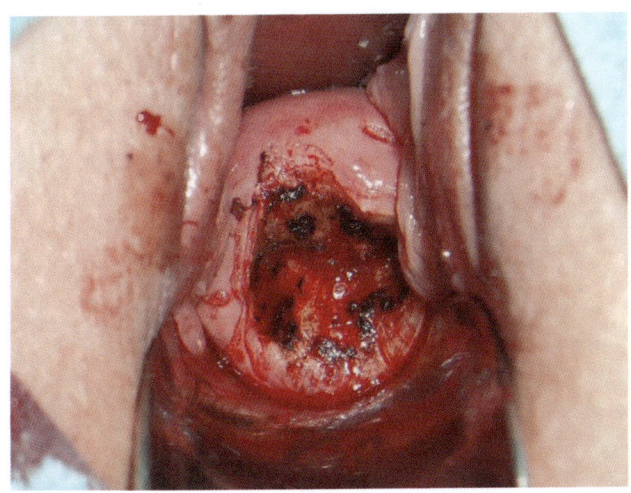

This is the image of a cervix immediately after a conization with an electrocautery loop. The section of cervix that has been removed is about the size of a medium strawberry. In cases of *in situ* cervical cancer, the tissue that is removed can be sent for pathological review to determine if there are clear margins.

Recall from Chapter 1 that HPV infects the immature cervical cells that reside in the deepest layer of the cervix [4]. The virus does not infect the mature cells at the surface; therefore, there must be an entry point for the virus to gain access. Anything that damages the surface of the cervix will expose these vulnerable cells to infection; this seems likely to include biopsies, LEEPs and conizations, where a very large area of immature cells is exposed. This would truly be disastrous if the modern medical treatment of CIN is resulting in disease recurrence and the persistence of HPV. Indeed, I suspect that this is the case because after treating this condition for twenty years, I have had a 99% success rate with all dysplasia, about a 90% rate of HPV elimination, and I rarely see HPV or dysplasia come back. When I contrast this to the aforementioned medical treatment stats, it seems that there is some problem with the conventional approach—namely that it doesn't work very well in more cases than is comfortable. Note that this is my *observation*. There aren't any studies comparing conventional treatment to my natural treatment. However, I have seen more cases than I would like of women who started with HPV and ended with a 6-10 year history of multiple LEEPs, biopsies and cones; I have never had this happen with a single patient that I've treated—even with these post-medical-debacle cases that I've cured.

Although most women tolerate a LEEP without apparent complications, there are reasons to avoid this procedure. A systematic review published in the *British Medical Journal* found that surgical treatment for CIN "was associated with a significantly increased risk of miscarriages in the second trimester"[56]. Other complications include infection, scarring and a narrowing or loss of the cervical canal causing infertility.

Additional reasons to avoid surgical procedures for the treatment of CIN are possible changes in sexual satisfaction and performance. I have had some women describe a decreased ability to orgasm, diminished intensity of orgasms, decreased clitoral sensitivity and/or discomfort with sex following LEEPs and conizations. These potential side effects are never disclosed to women undergoing surgical excisions because they are not recognized by the medical community to occur. **It's not that sexual side effects have been studied and found to not occur, but rather *they have not been studied at all.*** However, there are too many women reporting these symptoms in online chat forums to discount them out of hand. All the more frustrating (and infuriating), is that women experiencing side effects of this nature are brushed off by their doctors as neurotics and overly hypersensitive individuals. Whether sexual side effects are physical or emotional in nature doesn't matter because they are real for anyone experiencing them. Furthermore, mental and emotional states can modify sensory information coming into the brain, making fuzzy the arbitrary lines separating "physical" and "emotional". **This is an area that needs to be taken more seriously and research must be conducted to determine the incidence of sexual side effects to better inform women prior to submitting to excisional procedures.**

The Natural Treatment of HPV and Dysplasia

In contrast to conventional therapy, natural therapy is *ipso facto* holistic in its approach: it addresses the entire person in relation to the illness. In fact, HPV and CIN *necessitate* a holistic approach by the very fact that there are numerous circumstances that must be met for HPV to cause problems. In other words, there is a constellation of predisposing factors that allow HPV to transform a cell. **Removing abnormal cells with a scalpel does nothing to address why the abnormal cells occurred in the first place.** For a doctor to exclaim post-LEEP "Voila, you are cured my child", is absurd and wishful thinking. If possible, the most sensible approach to HPV and CIN is to address *all* of the factors involved; not only will this maximize the likelihood of elimination of the virus and precancerous cells, but will also decrease the chances of having reoccurrences.

My natural treatment for HPV and CIN consists of two parts: Oral treatment, which includes supplementation and diet; and **direct treatment**, which consists of the topical application of a solution that kills abnormal cells. The rationale for this approach is to selectively kill unhealthy, HPV-infected cells without affecting normal cells, and to facilitate the replacement of the dead cells with healthy, un-infected cells; and it accomplishes this with great success.

Oral Treatment

There are two parts to oral treatment: nutritional supplements and diet. I purposely didn't say "dietary *changes*" because it may be that you already have a great diet—one that is replete with a variety of vegetables and fruits—which can be all the more frustrating when you have a persistent HPV infection. Supplementation with vitamins, minerals and plant chemical extracts is simple pharmacology: the modification of bodily processes with ingested substances. The significance of these dietary nutrients is misunderstood, massively underappreciated, and the phrase "vitamins and minerals" has become cliché, but the fact is that you would get very sick and die in a short time without them. **The oral part of treatment is scientific: it is based almost entirely on research published in peer-reviewed medic al journals.** A primer on the subject of research should be instructive at this point.

"Peer-reviewed" medical journals enlist an advisory panel of experts and statisticians to review any research submitted for publication. For a paper to be published it must suffer the critical review of the advisory panel and if it is found to be unbiased and in accordance with the scientific method, without conflicts-of-interest, and its conclusions represent the results obtained accurately, it will be published. Once published, it is available for the scientific community to see via an "indexed" database such as *pubmed.gov*. PubMed is the research database of the National Library of Medicine and the National Institutes of Health. If a claim is made about anything and it is not backed by indexed research, for all intents and purposes, it does not exist. When a claim is made that is not referenced--in other words the indexed research source is not provided--I call that "talking out of one's ass". Personally, I try not to talk out of my ass, but if I do I will at least impart to the reader that my claim is either extrapolated from similar research or is based in scientific theory.

In Chapter 1, HPV characteristics were described that included the process of malignant transformation. Understand that an HPV infection is irrelevant, if not for the fact that the virus has the capacity, under certain conditions, to transform a normal cell into a cancerous one. Recall that in cervical cancer, as is the case with all cancer, the cell's internal machinery that is necessary for normal function is disrupted in a progressive fashion, and that several of these virally-induced mechanisms were described. They were the degradation of tumor suppression proteins, oxidative stress and the production of VEGF. **Appropriately, supplementation therapy consists of addressing all three of these processes; it consists of inhibiting malignant transformation.**

Oral Treatment to Inhibit Malignant Transformation

It is wise for all women with HPV to be proactive and treat an infection as soon as possible because we are unable to identify those women who will have problems with the virus. A "problem" refers to the development of a persistent infection and dysplasia. I consider even mild dysplasia a problem because it is not only the first step toward cancer, but also for the reason that it introduces emotion, fear and uncertainty into your life. Your doctor will continue to tell you not to worry about it, but if you do any investigation whatsoever you will likely discover the mismanaged horror cases online that started with CIN1 and ended with conization or hysterectomy. **So rather than play the risky waiting game, I advocate treatment as soon as you find out that you have any pap abnormality and/or HPV.** Incidentally, this would be the conventional approach if there was a specific FDA-approved drug or treatment vaccine for HPV.

Although I have found after twenty years of treating HPV and dysplasia that almost everyone with HPV focuses on eliminating the virus, the primary concern is, first and foremost, the prevention of cancer. Even CIN3 is a non-issue if it never turns into cancer. Thus, the most important facet of treatment is to prevent malignant transformation. No transformation, no cancer. Fortunately, we know something about this process and how to prevent it with oral supplementation.

There are numerous plant chemicals that have demonstrated the ability to protect or up-regulate tumor suppression activity, diminish oxidative stress and decrease VEGF. There are actually quite a few plant chemicals and supplements that can address each of the three main mechanisms of malignant transformation--so many in fact, that rather than recommend every single one, I instead use those which exhibit the ability to address all three *simultaneously*. All of the following phytochemicals have been shown to protect the tumor suppression proteins pRb and/or p53, diminish oxidative stress and decrease VEGF production (Please note that research references are provided):

- **DIM** (Di-indolyl methane) [57,58,59]: This is a chemical extract from brassica plants that include broccoli, cabbage, kale and Brussels sprouts. I-3-C (indole-3-

carbinol) is, in effect, the same as DIM. We've known that DIM reverses CIN since the 1990s. A 2009 study showed that DIM inhibits the progression from cervical dysplasia to cervical cancer as well as inhibit the development of E6/E7 oncogene induced cervical lesions [57]. And yes, it's great to eat lots of broccoli and cabbage but no; you're not going to get the amount of DIM that you want to treat CIN with diet alone.

- **Curcumin/Turmeric** [60,61,62,63]: Turmeric is a root spice that comes from the ginger family, *Zingiberaceae.* It is the dominant spice used in Indian curry that gives it its yellow color. Curcumin is the most active chemical constituent of the whole root, turmeric. Neither turmeric nor curcumin are well-absorbed and should be taken as a supplement in which piperine, bromelain or phosphatidyl choline is added to improve utilization. Curcumin is an outstanding anti-inflammatory, anti-cancer compound and there are studies that have used curcumin to potentiate prescription cancer drugs and radiation therapy while protecting healthy cells [64]. A 2011 study demonstrated that curcumin counteracts the stimulating effect of estrogen on HPV positive cells causing them to die [62] and it does this, at least in part, by inhibiting the E6 oncogene [63]. The turmeric supplement that I use is also combined with quercetin to maximize synergism.

- **EGCG** (epigallocatechin-3-gallate) [65,66,67]: EGCG is the most abundant catechin found in white tea, green tea and to a smaller extent, black tea. It is a powerful antioxidant that is also anti-cancer, anti-inflammatory and improves immunity. A 2009 study found that green tea was "suitable for prevention and treatment of cervical cancer" [65] and that in addition to diminishing oxidative stress, exerted some of its effects via a p53 mechanism [66]. A study in 2003 investigated green tea extract applied to the cervix and found it effective for treating cervical lesions [67]. Although this last study was intriguing because it used a vaginal suppository that could potentially be used as home-therapy, research conducted in 2014 attempted to reproduce these results and found green tea suppositories (polyphenon E) ineffective at treating CIN1 and HPV [68].

  Note to the reader: I have not used green tea vaginal suppositories in my practice, although I have had patients who have tried them. Most notable was a woman in Singapore who had used green tea as well as curcumin suppositories for the treatment of CIN3. The dysplasia did not resolve and she sought me out to do escharotic therapy. After 9 applications of bloodroot and zinc chloride the CIN was gone and she was HPV negative.

- **Resveratrol** [69,70,71]: Resveratrol is a polyphenol compound with strong antioxidant activity that is found in the skins of berries. There has been evidence that suggests an anti-aging and cardio-protective benefit, but there has been conflicting research and controversy in this regard; in the context of

HPV, we are just looking for inhibition of malignant transformation. A 2007 study showed that resveratrol suppresses E6- and E7-induced blood vessel growth in cervical cancer and "is a promising chemotherapeutic agent for human cervical cancer" [71]. Note that a cup of red grapes has only 1 mg of resveratrol content. Supplement dosages can exceed 1,000 mg (i.e. you'd have to eat 1,000 cups of grapes to equal what can be found in 1-2 pills).

- **Quercetin** [72,73,74]: Quercetin is a flavonoid found in many fruits and vegetables with the highest content found in cilantro, red onion and kale. Quercetin, like flavonoids in general, is an antioxidant with anti-inflammatory and anti-cancer properties. A 2010 study demonstrated that quercetin caused cervical cancer cells to die by a p53-dependent mechanism that was dose-dependent (more was better) and the authors suggested that quercetin was a "classic candidate for anticancer drug design" [72].

- **Alpha-lipoic acid** [75,76,77]: Alpha-lipoic acid (ALA), an organosulfur compound, is a very powerful and unique antioxidant in that it can be both fat-soluble and water-soluble. ALA has the ability to regenerate vitamin C and E and can potentiate the effects of glutathione and coenzyme Q10. It is also chelates or binds to heavy metals including mercury, cadmium, arsenic and lead, allowing them to be removed from the body. Although found in some foods, it took an estimated 10 tons of liver residue to isolate 30 mg of ALA when its chemical structure was first identified—you might want to take a supplement instead! Although there is no research on the effects of lipoic acid on cervical lesions and HPV, it is a unique and powerful free radical scavenger and there are hundreds of studies demonstrating its ability to inhibit malignant transformation.

- **Coenzyme Q10** [78,79,80,81]: Coenzyme Q10 (CoQ10), known also as ubiquinone, is a potent fat-soluble antioxidant that is necessary for proper energy production in every cell of the body. There are at least 12 genes necessary for the proper production of CoQ10 and a mutation in any one gene can lead to deficiency. The highest levels of dietary sources of CoQ10 are almost exclusively found in animal tissues, although olive, soybean and grape seed oils can have appreciable levels. The absorption of supplemental forms of CoQ10 can vary greatly and manufacturers have devised ways of increasing absorption, although this increases the cost dramatically; CoQ10 is one supplement for which you get what you pay. CoQ10 has been shown to inhibit cervical cancer cell growth as well as cause cancer cell death [78].

Do you appreciate the significance of what you've just read? **These supplements don't just treat one mechanism of malignant transformation but *all* mechanisms.** This is actually an amazing thing; it'd be like a blood pressure medication treating psoriasis and gout, all at the same time! The same plant compounds and supplements that favorably modulate tumor suppression genes are also great anti-oxidants that protect against oxidative damage and help block new blood vessel formation to developing tumors. This effect, where a chemic al has multiple actions at multiple locations, is known as *pleiotropism*.

Pleiotropism is the ability of a substance to act in more than one way and with entirely different mechanisms. Di-indolyl methane (DIM) is a great example of this: DIM, an extract from broccoli and cabbage, diminishes oxidative stress, protects the p53 tumor suppression proteins from degradation by the E6 HPV oncogene, blocks neovascularization and also can balance estrogen in a favorable way to eliminate dysplasia (we haven't discussed this part of treatment yet, but recall that estrogen is a cofactor in the development of CIN and cancer). Incidentally, DIM also acts *pleiotropically* to protect against breast [82] and ovarian cancer [83] as well, and even helps to prevent prostate cancer [82] in men (Recall that the only reason that you were not told about DIM is because it is not a patented, FDA-approved drug for the treatment of cervical abnormalities). This ability of naturally occurring plant substances is quite extraordinary and wonderful, but the wisdom and sensibility of their use in treating disease, including CIN and HPV, cannot be fully appreciated without discussing the effect of *combining* phytochemicals.

Beyond Pleiotropy: The Role of Synergism

When combined, plant chemicals often exhibit *synergistic* effects. Synergism refers to the creation of a whole that is greater than the sum of its parts. In the context of supplements, this means that the combined effect of two plant chemicals taken *together* exceeds the sum of the effects achieved with the supplements when taken *individually*. An April 2014 study examined the ability of curcumin and resveratrol to decrease lung tumors in mice. The researchers found that the combination of the two plant chemicals diminished tumors to a greater degree than what resulted by adding together the effects of curcumin and resveratrol when taken individually [84]. In other words, there was a synergistic effect which is best described as "one plus one equals three—not two". The researchers concluded that the **"The combination approach is the future of the war against cancer"**. This study sums up what scientists from around the globe are discovering: plant chemicals--and especially their combined effects--hold the key to future cancer therapy...and more effective therapy at that!

The *combination* to which the aforementioned study was referring is that of plant chemicals—not just curcumin and resveratrol, but others as well. There are so many phytochemicals that interact in synergistic ways, in fact, that the only practical way to capitalize on synergism and pleiotropy is to adopt a plant-based diet, one that is replete with a myriad of complex phytochemicals that interact in ways which we have just begun to appreciate.

The HPV Diet: Wholesale Pleiotropy and Synergism!

Many of us are confused about diet. Much of this confusion stems from what is sometimes contradictory information: vegans are telling us that veganism is the healthiest diet and that animal products will be the death of us, and Paleolithic advocates are telling us that carbohydrates and gluten are the devil and cause diabetes and a myriad of chronic degenerative diseases; and the fact is that there is research that supports both ends of the spectrum and there is research that refutes both ends of the spectrum. **Most of this confusion is artificial and created by zealots and capitalists.** The zealots would have you believe that an all-vegan diet is best, for example, but in reality their position is usually rooted in politics (i.e. they don't believe in killing animals), while the capitalists are rewarded by writing books that take one position or another—never in between, because moderation is boring. Extreme positions are controversial and controversy sells. Did you ever wonder how research could be so contradictory? The lay press will one day tell us that eating chocolate is good for you and on another day tell us that it is bad. I could give nearly countless examples of bad studies that are covered in the news, not because the information is useful, but more often because the study claims that prevailing beliefs are incorrect. The reality is much more straightforward, at least with regard to the topic at hand: **a plant-based diet has been shown to help eliminate HPV as well as increase the likelihood of getting rid of dysplasia.**

I define a plant-based diet as a diet characterized by the daily consumption of lots of vegetables and some fruits--and by my estimation corn and potatoes are not vegetables! The vegetables to which I refer are kale, arugula, parsley, collard greens, cabbage and dandelion. And the fruits to which I refer do not include bananas, which are high in sugar and low in antioxidants, but rather consist of the berries which are very high in the phytochemicals that are beneficial to immunity and to prevent malignant transformation. Additionally, my diet-of-choice does not include junk food or a reliance on carbohydrates that have been shown to inhibit the immune system as well as increase oxidative stress and free radicals. High fat and high carbohydrate meals have been shown to increase oxidative stress.

It is important to understand that the ultimate purpose of the "HPV Diet" is to consume large quantities of phytochemicals and antioxidants that inhibit malignant transformation as well as increase the ability of the immune system to eliminate HPV. To follow the HPV Diet is to engage in the wholesale acquisition of vast quantities of complex plant chemicals. It can be difficult to obtain pharmacologic levels of the phytochemicals outlined at the start of the "oral treatment" section with diet alone. However, the fruits and vegetables recommended in the HPV Diet contain a greater variety of phytochemicals and antioxidants than can be reasonably obtained via supplementation alone. The two go hand in hand: supplementation can provide the necessary quantities of specific nutrients in which research has demonstrated benefit, while diet can remove foods that impair immunity and at the same time provide a vast array of chemicals that act in synergistic and pleiotropic ways. In other words, the HPV

Diet forms the base of HPV and dysplasia treatment while supplementation provides key specific nutrients in amounts that are not practical to get with diet alone.

Contrary to the medical treatment guidelines for HPV and dysplasia there are many studies that have demonstrated a significant correlation with diet, dysplasia and HPV clearance. I have outlined some of the research below. While reading, please recognize that your doctor and the American Congress of Obstetricians and Gynecologists (ACOG) have chosen to ignore this fundamental association between diet and HPV. It seems apropos at this point to reference the ACOG Strategic Plan:

> "The Congress, as the premier organization for obstetricians and gynecologists and providers of women's health care, will provide the highest quality education worldwide, continuously improve health care for women through practice and research, lead advocacy for women's health care issues nationally and internationally, and provide excellent organizational support and services for our members."

Remember that your gynecologist follows guidelines created by this organization that chooses to ignore the research proving an association with diet, nutrition and HPV. Here are brief summaries of some of the research correlating diet and HPV:

> **"Higher levels of vegetable consumption were associated with a 54% decrease risk of HPV persistence. Also, a 56% reduction in HPV persistence risk was observed in women with the highest plasma cis-lycopene concentrations compared with the lowest..."** Cancer Epidemiology, Biomarkers & Prevention. "Vitamin A, Carotenoids, and Risk of Persistent Oncogenic Human Papilloma Infection", Vol 11, 876-884, September 2002.

Lycopene is a carotenoid compound that gives tomatoes and other red fruits and vegetables their color. Carotenoids include beta-carotene, lycopene, zeaxanthin, astaxanthin, and cryptoxanthin and are found in orange, red and yellow vegetables such as squash, carrots and sweet potatoes.

> **"Higher circulating levels of trans-zeaxanthin, total trans-lutein/zeaxanthin, cryptoxanthin, total trans-lycopene and cis-lycopene, carotene and total carotenoids were associated with a significant decrease in the clearance time of type-specific HPV infection, particularly during the early stages of infection (<or=120 days)."** Cancer Res. "Hawaii cohort study of serum micronutrient concentrations and clearance of incident oncogenic human papillomavirus infection of the cervix", 15;67(12):5987-96, June 2007.

What is especially interesting about this study is that blood micronutrient levels of carotenoids factored significantly into the ability to clear HPV, but only for recent infections (under 120 days); for infections greater than 120 days there was no significant correlation with dietary nutrients in this study. **The results of this study suggest that a proactive diet and nutritional support program should be implemented as soon as a HPV infection is detected.** This is one of many studies demonstrating the error in the "do-nothing" approach of conventional medicine. Remember this study and others like it when your doctor makes the false claim that "there is nothing you can do to get rid of HPV".

> **"Women with the unhealthiest dietary patterns were 3.5 times more likely to be diagnosed with CIN2+ than women with the healthiest dietary pattern."** *Cancer Prev Res.* "A dietary pattern associated with LINE-1 methylation alters the risk of developing cervical intraepithelial neoplasia", Mar;5(3):385-92, 2012.

Recall the association between folic acid, methylation, and the role that methylation has in preventing HPV infection as well as eliminating dysplasia. This study correlated dietary patterns and the degree of methylation of white blood cells (white blood cells can be used as a marker to measure methylation). Women who eat diets high in vegetables and fruits have higher amounts of methylation and a decreased likelihood of being diagnosed with CIN2 or worse.

> **"Women with supraphysiologic concentrations of plasma folate who also had sufficient plasma vitamin B12 had 70% lower odds of being diagnosed with CIN2+...."** *Cancer Prev Res.* "Lower risk of cervical intraepithelial neoplasia in women with high plasma folate and sufficient vitamin B12 in the post-folic acid fortification era", Jul;2(7):658-64, 2009.

"Supraphysiologic concentrations" denotes levels that are higher than average when measured in the blood. Note that dark green leafy vegetables have the highest folic acid content and that vitamin B12 is not found in plants but is only found in animal products; my recommendation is to obtain B12 supplementally.

> **"Women with higher plasma folate and higher HPV 16m or those with higher plasma vitamin B12 and higher HPV 16m were 75% and 60% less likely to be diagnosed with CIN2+, respectively."** *Cancer Prev Res.* "Folate and vitamin B12 may play a critical role in lowering the HPV 16 methylation associated risk of developing higher grades of CIN", Aug 21.pii: canprevres.0143, 2014.

I've described previously in Chapter 2 how methylation plays an important role in tumor suppression gene activity and cancer development. This study found that higher levels of folic acid and B12 resulted in more methylation of HPV 16 oncogenes, thereby *silencing* their activity and substantially decreasing the likelihood of developing moderate and severe dysplasia.

> **"The results of this study show an inverse association between serum antioxidant micronutrient concentrations and the risk of cervical neoplasia."** *Clin Chem Lab Med.* "Relationship of serum antioxidant micronutrients and sociodemographic factors to cervical neoplasia: a case-control study",47(8):1005-12, 2009.

The antioxidants that were measured in this study were beta-carotene, lycopene, zeaxanthin, lutein, vitamin A and vitamin E; the higher the levels of these antioxidants, the lower the risk of CIN. The researchers also found that cervical cancer was associated with older age and being overweight.

> **"Increasing concentrations of serum alpha- and gamma-tocopherols, and higher dietary intakes of dark green and deep yellow vegetables/fruit were associated with nearly 50% decreased risk of CIN3."** Int J Cancer. "Diet and serum micronutrients in relation to cervical neoplasia and cancer among low-income Brazilian women",Feb 1;126(3):703-14, 2010.

Alpha and gamma tocopherols are types of vitamin E that are fat-soluble antioxidants. Vitamin E is found in vegetable oils, nuts and seeds. Note that if taken as an oral supplement, vitamin E should be in the form of "mixed tocopherols" or "mixed tocotrienols" to avoid potential adverse effects associated with singular vitamin E such as "alpha-tocopherol" only.

Please note that although some of the aforementioned studies were measuring vitamins in the blood, these vitamins were correlated with dietary trends as opposed to supplementation, which is why these studies are discussed here with the HPV Diet.

Dr. Nick's Veggie Mix: Where the Wheels Hit the Pavement

With regard to the research pertaining to diet and HPV, it should be evident that there is consistency: a diet replete with dark green vegetables and yellow/orange fruits and vegetables decreases the likelihood of the dysplasia worsening, improves the chances of clearing the virus and increases the odds of diminishing or eliminating dysplasia.

- Does the research suggest that you should be vegan? No.

- Does the research indicate that you should be vegetarian? No.

- Does the research show that you should eat lots of fruits and vegetables? Yes!

In other words, you don't need to be militant or obsessive with your diet—you just need to eat more veggies and fruits. Unfortunately, this can be a struggle for many of us either because of the perception that we lack the time, lack the money, or simply because we've defined ourselves with the restrictive mantra "I don't like vegetables!" For those of us in this latter category remember your goal: the elimination of a nasty virus that can cause nasty problems.

Some of you may be vegetarian or vegan, which is fine, as long as you are eating lots of veggies and sufficient protein (too little protein impairs immunity; and incidentally, you're not going to get enough protein from vegetables). Many vegetarians and vegans, especially those that are young, actually do not typically have good diets. I call them "cheesatarians" and "carbotarians" because in their desire to restrict flesh they often trade lean meat for pasta, quinoa, rice and bread or they have cheese and dairy dominate their plate (or bowl: some vegetarians eat cereal for dinner!). Additionally, some eat too many fruits and too little greens. In any event, after twenty years of practice, I have seen more than my share of overweight, unhealthy vegans.

In my desire to eat more greens myself, I adopted the practice of making my own veggie mix. Besides the obvious benefit of eating more greens that contain hundreds of remarkable phytochemicals, the purpose of "Dr. Nick's Veggie Mix" is to make it *easy*; I am very busy and I don't have time to mess around with time-consuming preparation, and I expect that you may be in the same boat. It's also meant to get a large variety of greens on a daily basis and this is something with which even diligent vegetarians struggle. More variety of greens translates into more variety of plant chemicals--and it's the plant chemicals that are the goal (that is, in addition to fiber, vitamins and minerals).

—Dr. Nick's Veggie Mix—

Purchase the following greens—organic if possible. If the greens are healthy when obtained they will last about two weeks, so you may only need to do this twice per month.

- Kale (lancinate, purple or regular)

- Arugula (or spinach)

- Collard greens

- Dandelion

- Parsley

- Cilantro (omit if you're a cilantro hater!)

- Green or red cabbage

Wash the greens in a clean sink and cut into approximately 2" squares. I cleanse my sink with Soft Scrub Bleach to ensure that my greens don't pick up bacteria. I use a large salad spinner to remove as much water as possible, and then toss the greens into a paper grocery bag until I am finished. I then mix all of the greens and put into large plastic containers or gallon freezer bags. There is something about mixing them altogether that acts to preserve them; I think it is probably the parsley which takes a very long time to spoil.

Now you have little excuse to not eat these greens 1-3 times per day! If you haven't eaten these greens before, they are very bitter and it may take time getting used to them. As you will find in the meal recommendations below, you can eat them raw, cooked or drink them after blending with a juice extractor (i.e. a juicer that blends very thoroughly). Common extractors are the *Nutri Ninja™*, *Nutri Bullet™* and the *VitaMix™*. I do not recommend juicers that remove the fiber because the fiber is an important benefit of eating fruits and vegetables. You don't have to purchase an extractor, it just makes it simple, offers more variety of meals and snacks, and prevents mastication fatigue—these greens are fibrous and chewing them thoroughly is time-consuming and at times challenging!

Meal Recommendations* (choose one item under each meal/snack):

Breakfast (Always eat breakfast! Not eating is a physiologic stressor that will impair immunity and may cause weight gain):

- Dr. Nick's Veggies with 1-2 eggs*

- Small can of wild Pacific salmon w/ Dr. Nick's Veggies sautéed in olive oil

- Green Smoothie*

Snack:

- Fruit (other than banana)

- Nuts/Seeds (not more than 2 tablespoons)

- Green Smoothie*

- Unsweetened Greek yogurt w/ berries (frozen are easier, less expensive)

Lunch:

- Palm-sized portion lean meat (no skin, not breaded or deep fried), cooked or raw veggies, quinoa or rice (omit carbohydrates if you have PCOS or you're trying to lose weight)

- Greens and Beans*

- Salad: made with Dr. Nick's Veggie Mix, any other veggies you like, optional legumes, optional meat, tofu or tempeh, dressing (olive oil and/or vinegar; less than 2 tablespoons if trying to lose weight

Snack:

- Fruit (other than banana)

- Nuts/Seeds (no more than 2 tablespoons)

- Green Smoothie*

- Small serving of dark chocolate

Dinner:

- Salad (choose another option if you've already had salad this day): made with Dr. Nick's Veggie Mix, any other veggies you like, optional legumes, optional meat, tofu or tempeh, dressing (olive oil and/or vinegar; less than 2 tablespoons if trying to lose weight

- Palm-sized portion lean meat (no skin, not breaded or deep fried), sweet potato or squash, quinoa or rice (omit carbohydrates if you have PCOS or you're trying to lose weight)

- Soup and salad or sweet potato/squash

See Appendix B for recipes

One trick that you can utilize to improve your immune system function is to eat less—provided the food that you do eat is nutrient dense, like Dr. Nick's Veggie Mix. The more that you eat, the more free radicals that you produce, so intermittent fasting can be beneficial especially if you need to lose weight. One strategy is to not eat after 6 pm or to only have a green drink for your last meal of the day.

Oral Treatment to Improve Immunity

As described in Chapter 1, women with HIV/AIDS and those who are immunocompromised are at an increased likelihood of having viral persistence and worsening dysplasia. Like with most bodily functions, there is significant variability from person-to-person, and this is also the case with immunity. Even in healthy individuals there is tremendous variability in the immune system; we just don't have a very practical way to measure it, which is largely to do the fact that it is very complex. But most of us know people who get sick often and those who almost never get sick. Some of this variability is due to dietary factors, stress, amount of sleep and nutrition, but it is quite certain that there are also mutations (single nucleotide polymorphisms or "snips") that greatly affect immune status.

The most illuminating research in the context of immunity comes from studies that have verified the role of cell-mediated immunity in HPV clearance and the regression of severe dysplasia. A 2007 study in *Clinical Cancer Research* looked at T-helper cells in women with moderate to severe dysplasia caused by HPV16 [85]. The researchers found that women who quickly cleared the virus and eliminated the dysplasia had high numbers of T-helper cells that were specific to HPV16; conversely, women with persistent HGSIL and HPV16 did not have this targeted response by the immune system. **This is a very significant finding that supports treatment to increase cell-mediated immunity.**

In the absence of HIV/AIDS or other diseases that impair immunity, it doesn't really matter *why* your immune system is weak, just what to do about it. And if you're planning on heeding my dietary advice, you've already done much to improve immunity because what you put in your mouth from day-to-day is the most important consideration to make. It's quite simple, so I don't need to belabor the point: eat lots of greens and fruits and your immunity will improve; eat lots of sugar, soda, candy and simple carbohydrates and your immunity will suffer.

In addition to following the HPV diet, it is advisable to supplement with several compounds that have been shown to help clear the virus, or that have a theoretical basis in the absence of research. They are mushroom extracts, vitamin C, *astragalus* and *ashwagandha.*

Mushrooms: Mushroom extracts are my favorite supplement for increasing immunity. I've used them extensively since the late 1990s after I treated a patient with AIDS and HPV-related rectal cancer. After just two months of administering a blend of seven mushrooms, he had a tripling of his T-helper cells, much to the astonishment of his oncologist. Mushroom research has been ongoing for about 70 years with thousands of studies confirming this robust response—what can be a 200-300% increase in cell-mediated immunity! Although there is little research demonstrating that mushrooms eliminate HPV, there is vast research confirming that mushrooms may be the most effective means to improve immunity in general; thus, it is my contention that mushroom extracts serve an important role in the treatment of HPV and HPV-related conditions.

Recall that HPV impairs cell-mediated immunity at the site of infection; this characteristic allows it to "hide" and evade immune detection--the main reason HPV can be difficult to eliminate. It's a proven fact that individuals with impaired immunity are more likely to have persistent HPV and cervical cancer. Conversely, women with a robust immune response to HPV eliminate dysplasia and clear the virus more quickly and more effectively. Therefore, it is reasonable that anything that will improve immunity would be met with increased odds of eliminating the virus.

The chemical constituents responsible for the immune-stimulating function of mushrooms are known as glucans, complex polysaccharide (i.e. sugar) compounds divided into two types: alpha-glucans and beta-glucans. Although both alpha- and beta-glucans are found in a variety of fungi and yeast, most mushrooms are replete with one or the other, not usually both. For example, Maitake mushroom is high in beta-glucans while Shitake is high in alpha-glucans. This is why I prefer to use a mushroom blend as opposed to a singular extract: there are many different therapeutic mushrooms and one may improve one aspect of immunity while another works on a different aspect of immunity (i.e. the more the better!). A 2010 study found that topical beta-glucans increased the elimination rate of ASCUS, LSIL and CIN1 after 20 consecutive days of treatment [86].

AHCC (active hexose correlated compound) is recently a popular supplement prepared from cultured Shitake and *Basidiomycetes* mushrooms that is high in alpha-glucan *only*. Research published in February 2014 has shown that a combination of Maitake and Shitake out-performed AHCC in its ability to stimulate immune function [87]. As of January 2015, there is no published research demonstrating AHCC treats HPV or CIN and I am inclined to continue to use a blend of fungi (Reishi, Shitake, Caterpillar, Turkey Tail, Brazilian mushroom, Oyster mushroom, Maitake, Chaga mushroom and Baker's Yeast extract).

Vitamin C: Vitamin C, known chemically as ascorbic acid (AA), is a vitamin so commonly taken as to be rendered nearly cliché. Despite its banality, AA has been shown to increase cell-mediated immunity and prevent some types of cancer [88]. There are hundreds of medical studies attesting to this fact and to provide them is unnecessary in this context. Although strong evidence correlating vitamin C with HPV clearance is lacking, it is inexpensive and also has been shown to stabilize p53 and reduce oxidative stress [88]. I don't recommend AA for all of my patients, but it is advisable in cases of persistent HPV infection, moderate to severe CIN, older age and women who seem to have low immunity in general.

Astragalus: There are several thousand species of *Astragalus*--a plant with a long history of use in Chinese and Persian medicine. *Astragalus* has been found to be anti-inflammatory, anti-cancer, immune-stimulating, an antioxidant and it is antiviral [89]. This is another supplement that I don't use on a regular basis but has application for anyone struggling with weakened immunity.

Ashwagandha: *Withania somnifera,* known commonly as *ashwagandha,* is a plant used in Ayurvedic medicine that has a wide variety of health benefits. It has been shown to up-regulate tumor suppression proteins and diminish the activity of HPV oncogenes in human cervical cancer cells [90]. *Ashwagandha* is anti-inflammatory, antitumor, anti-stress, immune-stimulating and is an antioxidant that has rejuvenating properties [91].This is an especially useful supplement for those of us who are under a lot of stress, because stress impairs immune system function. A 2011 study found that *ashwagandha* combined with Maitake mushroom-derived glucans prevented stress-induced immune damage [92]. There are hundreds of studies attesting to the ability of *ashwagandha* to mitigate stress and improve immunity. If you are under chronic stress you may want to consider incorporating this extraordinary plant into your supplement regimen.

Oral Treatment: Additional Supplements

Folic Acid: As previously described, folate has an especially significant role in HPV infection, CIN and cervical cancer development. As early as 1966, a correlation has been made between folic acid deficiency and cervical cancer [13]. Women who have higher levels of circulating folic acid have a lower likelihood of becoming positive for HR-HPV infection, a decreased chance of having a persistent HR-HPV infection, and a greater likelihood of becoming HR-HPV negative [16]. Also, women who have HPV-16 and *low* levels of folic acid are significantly more likely to be diagnosed with CIN2 or greater dysplasia than are women with HPV-16 who have ***higher*** levels of folic acid [17].

Unfortunately, many women have a mutation in the enzyme that allows folic acid to do what it is supposed to do, which is to methylate tumor suppression genes and oncogenes, turning some on and others off. Although we don't understand this process fully, we nonetheless know that this function of methylated folic acid is extremely important in the context of dysplasia and cervical cancer. You can be tested for the MTHFR (methylene tetrahydrofolate reductase) mutation with a blood sample; however, I don't typically perform this test because the treatment is quite simple: take *methylated* folate as opposed to *regular* folate. The two can be distinguished quite easily by looking at the supplement label; if it doesn't say "methyl tetrahydrofolate" then it's regular folic acid and you should not be taking it.

Multivitamin: The benefit of a good multivitamin is that it provides many vitamins, minerals and plant chemicals that may help with HPV and CIN, but don't have enough evidence to justify taking as separate supplements. I like to be cost-effective, using as little therapy as possible to eliminate HPV and dysplasia; so rather than give patients twenty different supplements, I prefer to use the supplements that have the most evidentiary support, so I prescribe a multivitamin to obtain everything else that might be beneficial in one pill. For example, there is some limited research showing that vitamin A, beta-carotene and vitamin E are useful to treat CIN, but not enough to justify taking each one individually as a distinct supplement; but nor do I want to neglect a nutrient that may be beneficial, so my solution is to use a good multivitamin.

A "good" multi should have methyl folate and a pharmacologic level of additional phytochemicals. As previously discussed, plant chemicals are synergistic, so the greater the variety the greater the benefit; however, they must be at a high enough dose to exert a physiologic or epigenetic change. An additional benefit of more phytochemicals is that they are also great antioxidants: my multi has an ORAC value of 25,000 because it contains 400 mg of a phytonutrient blend. ORAC (oxygen radical absorption capacity) is the standardized measurement of the ability of a substance to eliminate free radicals. An ORAC of 25,000 is insanely high and has been proven to stabilize and protect DNA. **A**

2010 study found that women who took multivitamins had lower HPV viral loads and had a significantly decreased frequency of CIN [93].

Probiotics: Research in the past 5-10 years has solidified the importance of gut bacteria with regard to human health—especially when it comes to a healthy, robust immune function. You actually have more bacteria residing in your intestine than you have human cells in your entire body and these residents are critical to normal health. A 2013 study found that probiotic users had double the chance of clearing dysplasia when compared to non-users [94]. A 2012 study showed that a Bifidobacterium species decreased the activity of the E6 and E7 HPV oncogenes [95].

My probiotic-of-choice is spore-based. Some bacteria are able to go into a dormant stage, known as a spore that is extremely resistant to everything that would normally kill most bacteria. When ingested, spore bacteria survive the stomach intact and "come alive" further down the intestine and start doing a number of cool things. One of the species of bacteria that I use is *Bacillus indicus*, an organism that will produce carotenoid compounds that will be absorbed directly thru the intestinal wall. Carotenoid compounds such as lutein, beta-carotene, astaxanthin, lycopene and zeaxanthin have been correlated with dysplasia improvement.

Vitamin D: Vitamin D deficiency is epidemic and if you are not taking it in the form of a supplement you are very likely deficient as well. Like other hormones in the body, vitamin D does many things and has been shown to be anti-cancer, immune stimulating and anti-inflammatory. Deficiency is correlated with over thirty diseases including diabetes, polycystic ovarian syndrome, depression and cancer. As of January 2015 there isn't any research that correlates oral vitamin D supplementation with HPV or CIN; however, there is a January 2014 study that demonstrated that vitamin D vaginal suppositories could help to eliminate CIN1 [96]. Despite a lack of research regarding oral vitamin D and CIN, deficiency must be addressed; I recommend either to have blood levels tested (vitamin D should be 50-70ng/mL) or to take 3,000-5,000 IU per day with food.

A Final Word on Research and Data Interpretation: An Omission of Facts

It is likely that at some point you were told by your doctor that there is no treatment for CIN other than surgery; or you were told that there is nothing you can do to eliminate HPV. As I've revealed to you there are many factors that relate to HPV persistence and research has provided insight regarding sensible treatment. **Despite this, you may still harbor doubt regarding natural treatment and this is only due to the fact that your gynecologist has not made the recommendations that I have made.** Who should you trust? It's actually more about *what* to trust. Trust the research. Remember that your doctor is compelled to follow the ACOG guidelines—a written standard-of-care that ignores much of what is known about HPV. Although part of the reason for this is the cost-prohibitive nature of getting FDA approval for a supplement that anyone can sell, another part is the lack of a type of research that carries the most weight clinically: randomized, double-blinded placebo-controlled human trials.

Known as a RCT (randomized controlled trial) for short, this gold standard in research carries the most weight in determining if one thing is related to another thing. For example, if I wanted to see if my supplement treatment for CIN is more effective than doing nothing, I'd have to procure two large groups of women—large enough so that there would be statistical significance at the end of it all. The women would have to be randomly assigned to one group getting treatment and to one group not getting treatment. However, for the study to be valid all of the women in both groups and the treating doctors could not know who is getting the real treatment and who is getting the placebo or "sham" treatment. In other words, none of the women can know who is getting the treatment supplements and who is getting pills with nothing in them. RCT's are great to have; the problem is getting funding. Nobody has ever performed a RCT on my oral treatment regimen because of the cost as well as the entity that stands to gain financially, which is no one that matters (supplement companies don't matter; big pharma does). To add further difficulty is the fact that an IRB (institutional review board) will not approve a study if it may result in the harm of a person.

For example, if I wanted to perform a study investigating the use of curcumin in treating cervical cancer I would not be able to do it. It would be a violation of the *Nuremberg Code*, a set of research ethics adopted worldwide after Nazi human experiment atrocities following World War II. I wouldn't be allowed to do it, because by using curcumin as cervical cancer treatment alone, I would be withholding accepted medical treatment that may be to the detriment of the study participants. For this reason, most research performed on potential drugs (this includes plant "drugs") is done initially in the laboratory setting and later on animals. Human subjects are usually the last to be experimented upon.

Although there are certainly human clinical trials investigating individual supplements, there are few that look at *combinations* of supplements. This is unfortunate because natural medicine treatment seldom relies on one thing; rather, natural medicine is integrative, using everything and anything that is reasonable to accomplish a treatment goal. This lack of RCT's presents a problem for natural medicine advocates. **However, it's hypocritical for critics of natural medicine to exclaim "where is the research?" when the problem is "where is the money?"** No money no research. Fortunately, there is enough laboratory and animal research to make extrapolations and arrive at what are reasonable conclusions.

I describe this extrapolation as "connecting the dots". For example, if human clinical trials using a novel plant chemical are lacking, but numerous studies on cultured cervical cell lines show an inhibition of malignant transformation, and research in animals demonstrate the same thing, it would seem very likely that the same effect would occur in humans. In other words, connect the dots! Although a human trial would be nice, if the prevailing research that is available is suggesting a benefit, I'm inclined to recommend the substance provided there is little or no risk.

Take curcumin for example: studies have shown that it can inhibit cervical cancer in a laboratory setting (when I refer to a "laboratory setting" I am referring to the effect a substance has on cells that are grown in a dish or *in vitro*. *In vitro* is Latin for "in the glass"; this is in contrast to *in vivo* which is Latin for "in the living"). So again, curcumin inhibits the growth of cervical cancer cells *in vitro*; it also inhibits HPV, protects p53 tumor suppression proteins, diminishes oxidative stress, inhibits VEGF and decreases inflammation. Curcumin helps to prevent all of the things that HPV does to cause cervical cancer, and yet there are no *human* trials showing that it prevents cervical cancer or dysplasia. So does a rational person cross his or her fingers, hoping for miracle-funding to conduct a human trial to *prove* that curcumin is effective? Your conventional doctor will very likely say yes, but I say of course not! I started using curcumin as part of my escharotic treatment as well as the oral treatment for cervical dysplasia in 2013. I did this because I noticed the direction of the prevailing research and made an extrapolation: I connected the dots. And the side effects of curcumin? Well, it has been shown to decrease pain and inflammation, improve the vascular system, and help prevent just about every other known cancer--that's good enough for me!

The "omission of facts" heading to this section refers to the untruth spoken by your doctor when you were told that there is nothing to do for HPV and no other treatment for CIN. On the one hand, your doctor is mostly correct that there aren't many RCT's supporting HPV treatment (there are some but they are conveniently disregarded); but your doctor is omitting the facts at the same time because there is vast research that supports it in the form of animal and laboratory studies. **Of course another likely possibility is that your doctor is ignorant of the research and has mistakenly concluded that there is no other treatment because the ACOG guidelines say so. In any event, your doctor has failed to properly inform you.**

However, this extrapolation is not fool proof. For example, green tea extract (epigallocatechin-3-gallate or EGCG) has a great deal of research demonstrating a likely benefit with regard to HPV and dysplasia. A 2009 study demonstrated that green tea extract inhibited the growth of cervical cancer cells *in vitro*. In effect, the green tea caused the cancer cells to stop growing and die, which is exciting to say the least. The researchers concluded that "EGCG may be suitable for prevention and treatment of cervical cancer." [65] However, a human clinical trial that was published in 2014 found no benefit to taking green tea extract. The study consisted of 98 women taking either green tea extract or a placebo, and it was found that after 4 months of taking 800mg of green tea daily, the study participants did not clear HPV nor eliminate dysplasia any better than the placebo group [68]. I can claim that four months was not long enough intervention or that green tea works better with more severe dysplasia, but the fact remains that this trial—the only trial looking at green tea with regard to HPV and mild dysplasia *in humans*—discerned no benefit!

Despite the fact that green tea by itself may not cure HPV or mild dysplasia, I still recommend it based on the strong likelihood that there is a synergistic effect of green tea extract when used in combination with other phytochemicals and a plant-based diet. Refer back to the April 2014 study that proclaimed that the future of cancer therapy is combination therapy, not single drug therapy. You see, this study only looked at green tea *by itself*, an unrealistic endeavor since a natural medicine physician would never recommend green tea as the sole treatment for CIN.

Ever since the birth of pharmacology in the mid-1850s, the medical community has been obsessed with a "one drug, one effect" mentality that pervades medicine to this day: the colloquial "magic bullet". Research has maintained this agenda to this very day. Those of you who are astute may be asking yourselves "Well why the heck don't they do human trials using *everything* that appears to inhibit HPV and dysplasia *at the same time*!?" Ah, but you see, you can't patent a combination of substances—or at least it's never been done. Remember that ultimately what drives research and FDA-approval of a drug is the bottom line. No money, no drug. No pharmaceutical company is going to invest in getting approval of something that can be purchased over-the-counter. And with no FDA approval there will be no change in the standard-of-care and subsequently, no recommendation by your doctor.

Summary of Oral Treatment

1) **Eat a plant-based diet replete with low-carbohydrate vegetables and fruits.** Concentrate on dark green leafy vegetables (Dr. Nick's Veggie Mix) as well as yellow-, red- and orange-colored veggies. The best fruits are the berries. Consider using a nutrient extractor (juicer) to simplify eating large quantities of veggies and fruits.

2) **Supplement with the following:**

   a. **DIM or I3C:** 200-300 mg two times per day with food.

   b. **Curcumin/Turmeric:** 500 mg two times per day with food.

   c. **EGCG/Green Tea Extract:** 100 mg two times per day with food.

   d. **Resveratrol/Red Wine Extract:** 50-100 mg two times per day with food.

   e. **Quercetin:** 100 mg two times per day with food.

   f. **Alpha-Lipoic Acid:** 100 mg two times per day with food.

   g. **Co-enzyme Q10:** 100 mg per day with food.

h. **Mushrooms:** 500-750 mg per day with food. Should contain at least 6 different mushrooms and standardized glucans.

i. **Vitamin C:** 500 mg two times per day. Take 1000 mg two times per day if you are post-menopausal or have weakened immunity.

j. **Astragalus:** Dose depends upon whether liquid or capsule. Take two times per day if you are post-menopausal or have weakened immunity.

k. **Ashwagandha:** Dose depends upon whether liquid or capsule. Take two times per day if you are under high stress or have weakened immunity.

l. **Methyl-Folate (5-methyl tetrahydrofolate):** 2000 mcg per day with food. Do not take folate that is not methylated; you cannot obtain methyl-folate from foods or from a "whole food" supplement. It is better to take with B2, B6 and B12 because these additional vitamins are also involved with bodily methylation.

m. **Multi-Vitamin:** Once per day with food. Do not take a cheap multi-vitamin. Do not take if it doesn't contain methyl-folate. If it says "folate" or "folic acid" it is *not* methylated. I prefer to use a multi that also contains a 400 mg "phytonutrient blend" of citrus bioflavonoids, green coffee bean, pomegranate, green tea, grape seed, bitter melon and a handful of other plants with high polyphenol and catechin content. This addition has been proven to protect your DNA from damage with an ORAC value of 25,000.

n. **Probiotics:** My probiotic-of-choice is a bacillus spore. A spore is a highly protective form of some bacteria that can survive incredibly harsh conditions. Even boiling spores will not kill them. Spore-producing bacillus organisms are the ideal probiotic because they can survive the stomach acid 100% intact and populate the lower intestine where they do cool things. Bacillus spores are found in the digestive tracts of all organisms on the planet, confirming their importance as a commonly ingested bacterium. The spore-based probiotic that I recommend has five different bacillus organisms including *Bacillus indicus,* which produces carotenoid compounds when it reaches the intestine. Carotenoid compounds include beta-carotene, lutein, astaxanthin and zeaxanthin—all of which have been shown to help eliminate HPV and CIN. The benefit of intestinal production of carotenoids is that they are not destroyed by stomach acid which happens with ingested carotenoid supplements.

I recommend two capsules containing at least 4 billion spores per day with food.

o. **Vitamin D:** Take whatever amount will total 3,000-5,000 IU of vitamin D per day when combined with other sources of vitamin D (such as your multi, etc.). Always take with food. If there is any uncertainty regarding the right amount for you, have your blood levels checked; you want to be at 50-70 ng/mL. If you think that you get enough vitamin D from sun exposure, you are likely wrong--have your levels checked.

If this seems like a lot of supplements to take, try finding ones that contains multiple compounds. For example, I have a supplement that contains vitamin A, vitamin C, selenium, alpha-lipoic acid, green tea, quercetin, and red wine extract—the equivalent of five of the recommended HPV supplements, all in one pill. Know also that this treatment regimen is not forever—it should be followed until your pap is normal and/or the HPV is gone, then you can eliminate many of the supplements, continuing with vitamin D and a good multivitamin containing methyl folate. This multi and vitamin D should be taken *forever*.

Chapter 4-Direct Treatment: Painting a Target on HPV and Dysplasia

Previously, I revealed the importance of diet and nutritional supplements in the treatment of CIN and HPV along with the supportive research. This research has been completely and utterly ignored by mainstream medicine. The failure to capitalize on decades of research substantiating the critical role that diet and nutrition plays in the elimination of HPV and dysplasia is egregious on the part of mainstream medicine and reflects a reductionist preoccupation with surgery and a magic bullet drug-mentality. **The conventional medical approach to HPV and dysplasia is likely to harm you.**

We are now going to embark on the second part of my natural treatment which is the direct application of a dysplasia- and HPV-killing-solution to the uterine cervix. **Termed an *escharotic*, this solution is comprised of bloodroot (*Sanguinaria canadensis*) and zinc chloride (ZnCl).** An escharotic is a substance that has the potential to destroy tissue causing a scab to form; this may sound a bit scary, but the acetic acid that is applied to the cervix during a colposcopic examination can also destroy tissue if undiluted or if left on for too long. **The goal of using an escharotic solution is to *selectively* kill HPV-infected cells and dysplastic cells with minimal or no damage to healthy, non-infected cells of the cervix.**

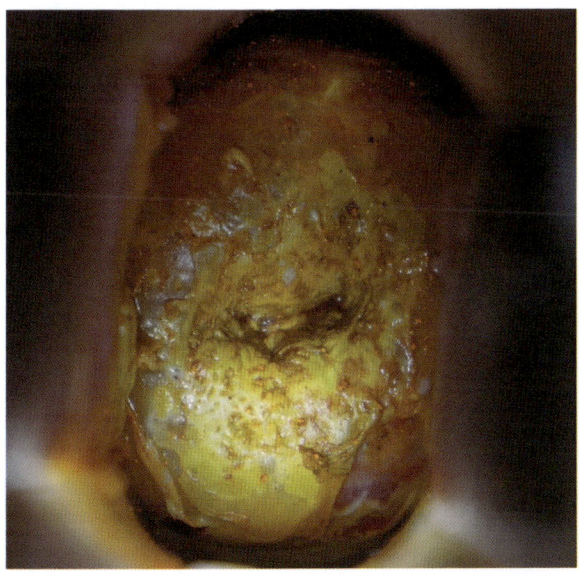

This image demonstrates the formation of an eschar, or scab, the day after one application of escharotic solution in a 31-year old with CIN3. Note that dead cells are in the process of sloughing or peeling off. The area affected can vary dramatically; in this case the area is quite large.

It is important to understand and appreciate that *Sanguinaria* does not indiscriminately destroy cells like a chemical acid. It preferentially targets abnormal cells due to their diminished capacity for membrane stressors that upset ionic gradients. Ion gradients and electrical charges across cell membranes are necessary for the cell to perform its functions—necessary for life itself. As an HPV-infected cell is undergoing the process of malignant transformation, there are alterations in the cell membrane that make it more susceptible to external assault than normal, uninfected cells. The escharotic solution capitalizes on this phenomenon.

The Mechanism of Escharotic Therapy: Sodium-Potassium Pump Inhibition

When you visualize the cervix microscopically, there is a layer of cells on the surface that forms a protective skin of sorts. Each one of these cells is like a tiny factory with specific functions to perform. One of these functions is to move sodium out of the cell while coupling this with the active movement of potassium into the cell. In order to accomplish this task, there are transport channels that provide a passage through the outer membrane of the cell. These passages are known as *Sodium-Potassium Pumps* (Na-K pumps). The ultimate purpose of Na-K pumps is to create an electro-chemical gradient—in effect, an electrical charge—across the cell membrane for the purpose of performing other types of necessary tasks. Without this electrical gradient the cell is dead.

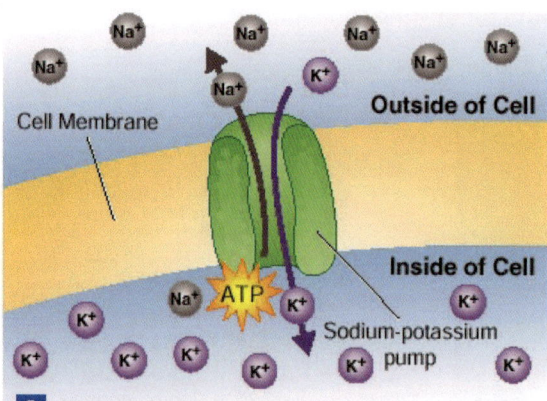

This illustration depicts a cell membrane which has a negative charge on the inside of the cell. The maintenance of this charge is the duty of sodium/potassium pumps. Loss of pump activity will result in the cell losing its charge and death of the cell.

A A protein pump in the neuron cell membrane uses the energy of ATP to pump Na+ out of the cell, and at the same time to pump K+ in.

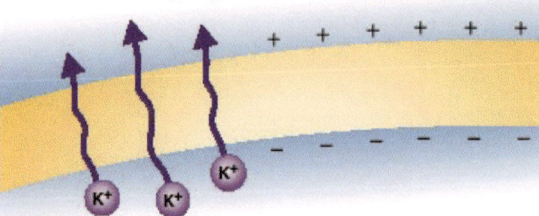

B The cell membrane is leakier to K+ than it is to Na+. Because more positive charges leak out of the cell than leak in, the inside of the cell becomes negatively charged with respect to the outside.

In the 1970s, research led to the postulation that malignant and pre-malignant cells become more leaky with regard to sodium and potassium [97,98]. Known as the "leakage theory" of cancer, this increase in the passage of sodium and potassium is due to increased membrane permeability that necessitates an increase in Na-K pump activity; the result is that more potassium is on the inside of the cell which is favorable for abnormal cell growth and division (i.e. cancer). In other words, pre-cancerous and cancerous cells prefer more potassium inside of the cell than exists in a normal cell, and this is accomplished with increased Na-K pump activity. The increase in pump activity can be as much as five times that of a healthy cell [99].

The relationship between drugs that decrease Na-K pump function and cancer inhibition was stumbled upon accidentally when analyzing data from patients taking medications for cardiac failure. Researchers discovered that these patients who were taking pump inhibitors, such as digoxin, had diminished incidence of numerous types of cancer [100-106]. It has been discovered that bloodroot, the primary ingredient in the escharotic solution, is also a sodium-potassium pump inhibitor [107].

There were twenty studies published from 2013-2014 demonstrating the ability of sanguinarine (the active alkaloid chemical extracted from bloodroot) to kill a variety of cancers including cervical cancer [108]. By inhibiting the sodium-potassium pump, exposure of cells to bloodroot causes them to lose potassium from the inside of the cell [109]. Recall that pre-cancerous and cancerous cells are already leaking potassium (the leakage theory) and with bloodroot exposure are leaking even more, a condition which is intolerable to these abnormal cells; thus, they die.

Another interesting mechanism by which bloodroot may destroy cancer is by uncoupling glucose transport through the cancer cell membrane. Glucose (sugar) transport into the cell is an active phenomenon which requires energy to occur. One way for this transport to happen is by coupling this movement of sugar with sodium, whose concentration is greater on the outside of the cell due to the activities of Na-K pumps. In effect, sodium wants to go back into the cell and sugar hitches a ride. By inhibiting pumps, sanguinarine will cause the concentration of sodium on the outside of the cell to diminish, thereby decreasing the concentration gradient across the cell membrane. This makes it difficult for sugar to get into the cell to fuel cancer activities; thus, the cell dies.

To summarize, the selectivity of the escharotic solution is due to the fact that healthy cells with normal pump activity can withstand limited solution exposure. Cells undergoing malignant transformation—in other words, HPV-infected cells and CIN— have ever-increasing expression of pumps due to increased metabolic needs and potassium leakage; thus, they are more reliant on sustained pump activity and are more likely to die with escharotic exposure [110-113]. *Note: it is not advisable to take bloodroot orally because it can be toxic and because it is modified inside the body rendering it less effective [107]). Also, it is not advisable to use an escharotic paste on the external surface of the body where it may be left on for days while it damages tissue—sometimes causing horrific scarring. The claim that salves or pastes can be used externally to identify and kill internal cancers lacks scientific credibility, is dangerous, and should never be attempted.*

The Mechanism of Escharotic Therapy: Painting a Target on HPV

The escharotic solution has an affinity for HPV-infected and dysplastic cells, clearly causing their destruction as demonstrated with the formation of an eschar or scab. This creates localized inflammation and an immune response ensues. Within hours of cervical cell destruction and inflammation, blood-borne white blood cells, known as monocytes, migrate to the site of destruction and transform into tissue macrophages. These macrophages, known as dendritic cells, gobble up dead cells on the cervix, in the endocervical canal and on the vaginal walls. What is brilliant is that when dendritic cells encounter foreign viruses, they move the viruses to their surface and then "present" this invader to other immune system cells, such as T helper cells. T helper cells are considered the commanders-in-chief of cell-mediated immunity, critical for a robust immune response.

Recall from Chapter 1 that HPV inhibits cell-mediated immunity in its attempt to 'hide" from the immune system. Therefore, in a strategic move against the virus, T helper cells are called to action by HPV-presenting dendritic cells. In effect, the dendritic cells marshal the troops to go after any and all HPV-infected cells in the region--they cause a localized immune frenzy at the site of HPV infection. Therefore, escharotic treatment does not simply consist of tissue destruction at the hands of a caustic solution, but the selective targeting of abnormal cells by the immune system. **The escharotic treatment is "painting a target" on HPV and CIN.** Thus, the mechanism-of-action with escharotic therapy is at least two-fold: abnormal cell destruction by sodium-potassium pump inhibition and by the facilitation of a highly selective immune system targeting of the virus.

It is my contention that escharotic therapy is superior to a LEEP. A LEEP is an arbitrary removal of cervical tissue with little regard for healthy versus diseased tissue. It's comparable to removing an entire foot due to gangrene of one toe. Nor does a LEEP elicit a sustained inflammation or a targeted immune attack as in the case with an 8-12 week course of escharotics. Furthermore, escharotic therapy does not cause scarring of the cervix nor result in the increased risk of pre-term labor as is the case with surgical procedures. Additionally, escharotic intervention does not require downtime for recovery as is the case with surgical excision; my patients are in and out of my office in 15 minutes without restrictions in activities.

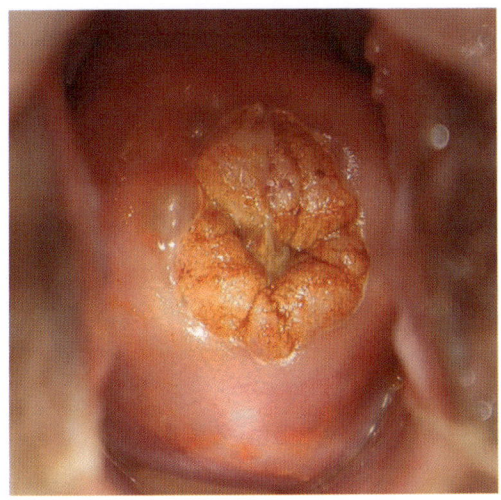 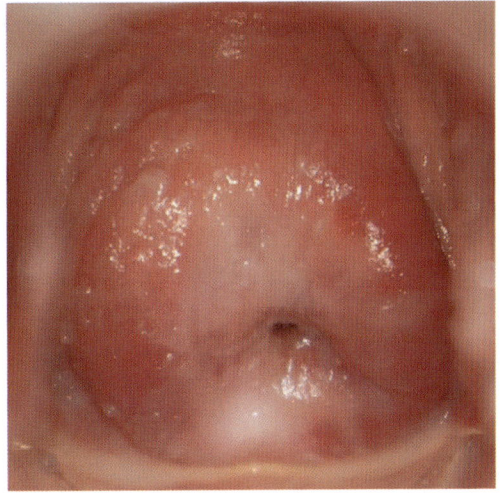

This is the cervix of a 35-year old woman with high-risk HPV and CIN2. The image to the left is after the initial escharotic application. Note that there are cysts at the edge of the lesion at 10:00 and 11:00, indicating chronic cervicitis (inflammation). The image to the right is at the completion of treatment. There has been a dramatic remodeling of the surface with the elimination of HPV, CIN and cervicitis.

How Escharotic Therapy is Performed

The treatment protocol for the administration of escharotic therapy is simple: the patient assumes a position on an examination table with her feet in the stirrups (just like when having a pap), the cervix is visualized with the assistance of a speculum, and **the escharotic solution is "painted" onto the cervix.** For the sake of efficiency, I have evolved my therapy to use a disposable pipette to bathe the entire cervix as opposed to using cotton swabs. Using a pipette also allows me to treat the entire vaginal canal very easily; this is to minimize missing areas of dysplasia that may be hidden on the walls as well as to maximize the likelihood of killing any and all cells harboring the virus. I always apply the solution to the endocervical canal regardless of whether there is known endocervical involvement as identified with the endocervical curettage component--or "ECC" portion--of a colposcopically-directed biopsy.

Once the solution has been in place for 60-90 seconds it is removed. For about the first fifteen years of providing this therapy, I would end the treatment by putting a tampon against the cervix that had been covered in a salve containing goldenseal, Thuja, tea tree oil and bitter orange. This tampon was left in place for 12-24 hours and removed by the patient. In recent years I have used it less often because it doesn't seem to make a difference in the treatment outcome.

The cervix should be treated with escharotic solution once per week until there is no longer evidence of dysplasia. The exception to this frequency of treatment are women travelling a great distance to see me; in these cases I may opt to perform two treatments two days in a row and do that 1-2 times per month. This allows for less travelling and minimizes the cost. **Because the solution stains abnormal and HPV-infected cells a white color, the regression of dysplasia can be witnessed and the treatment modified accordingly.** I always take before and after images with every treatment so that I can have a discussion with the patient regarding how it's coming along. The total time for each treatment, including discussing the before and after cervical images, is about 15 minutes.

Vaginal Suppositories

There are a variety of vaginal suppositories that can be self-administered in the privacy of your home. Although I have known women who have made suppositories themselves, many are available to order online and include "vag pack", green tea, curcumin, tea tree oil and other essential oil suppositories. As in the case of the pack described above, I use these less often than in past years because I have not found them to be particularly effective. Additionally, I have consulted with many women internationally who have attempted to use suppositories for CIN without satisfactory results. I have never come across anyone who has eliminated moderate or severe dysplasia with these alone, and I do not recommend them except in cases of recently diagnosed mild dysplasia where the alternative is to watch and wait, and when the use of escharotics are not available.

There are some exceptions to my rule regarding suppositories: I sometimes use them with women travelling to my office from afar; and I use them in cases involving comorbidities such as cervicitis (inflammation) and imbalances in vaginal bacteria. My rationale in the former scenario is that I want to use everything and anything that is going to get the job done as quickly as possible, because women travelling from a distance are investing significant money for the flight and lodging. In these cases I tend to err on overtreatment for the sake of keeping the number of trips to Chicago at a minimum.

Comorbidities, which are disease conditions *in addition* to HPV and CIN, include cervicitis and bacterial imbalances and should be treated in their own right. Cervicitis is inflammation of the cervix that may be due to a low-grade infection.

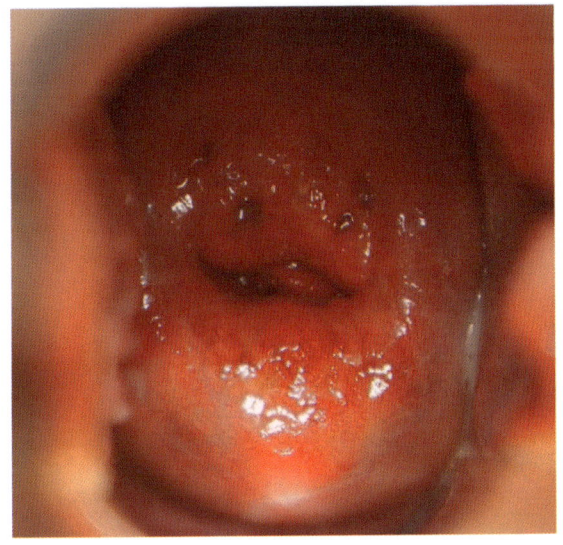

This image demonstrates cervicitis, a chronic inflammation of the cervix. Note the "pits" on the upper part of the cervix which are remnants of Nabothian cysts—a hallmark of chronic cervicitis. There is also a polyp in the canal that was eliminated with escharotic therapy. This patient also had CIN3 in the canal and outer cervix that was eliminated after 11 escharotic applications.

A 2014 study found that 98.7% of women with cervicitis had a HPV infection [114]; whether the HPV contributed to the cervicitis or whether cervicitis increases the HPV infection rate is unclear. In these cases, I may use a suppository that is anti-bacterial such as goldenseal, tea tree oil or other essential oils. I have been using curcumin suppositories for this condition more recently because it is an outstanding anti-inflammatory compound and because it has also been shown to inhibit HPV and CIN with a topical application in several studies [115,116,117].

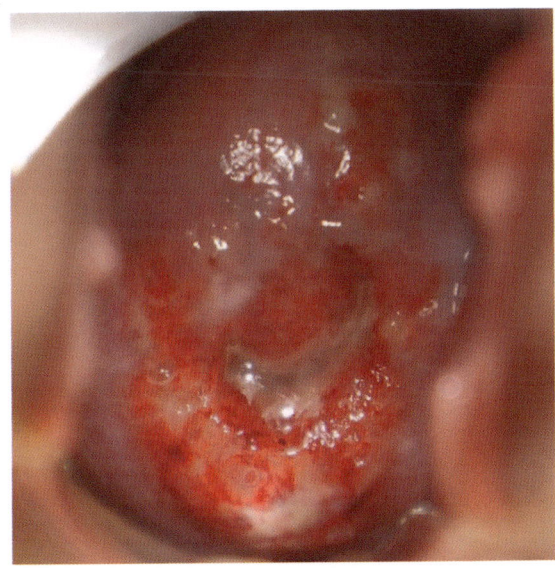

Image 1: This is the cervix of a 42-year old woman who had moderate dysplasia on the outer cervix and mild dysplasia in the canal. She was responding slowly because her case was made more difficult by concurrent severe cervicitis identified by the redness and the Nabothian cysts (pimple-like structures). At this point, I decided to add curcumin to the escharotic solution based on research demonstrating the anti-inflammatory effects of curcumin.

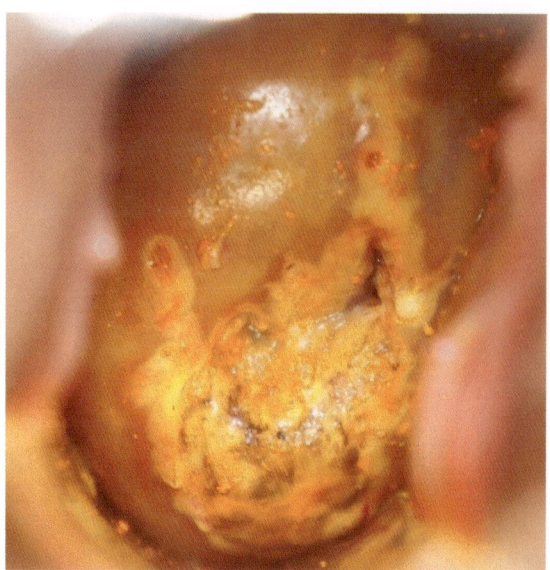

Image 2: This is the same patient after applying the escharotic solution combined with curcumin. Note that the white/yellow areas are staining attributable to dysplasia and/or inflammation. This was her eighth escharotic application but the first with the addition of curcumin.

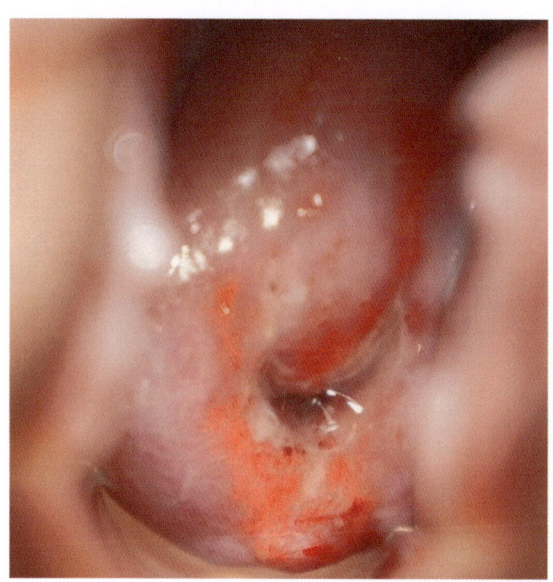

Image 3: This picture was taken two weeks after image 2. Note that the redness and cysts are considerably improved as compared to image 1.

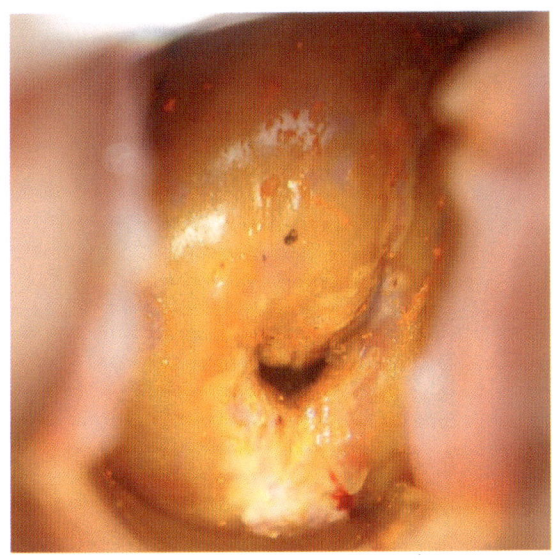

Image 4: This image was taken on the same day as image 3 after the application of escharotic with curcumin. The area staining is substantially smaller than in image 2. For a case that was slow to improve (I had already done 7 applications at the time of image 1), one treatment with curcumin resulted in a 50% reduction in the size of the lesion. It was this case that has prompted me to use curcumin in all subsequent cases.

Imbalances in the vaginal flora are common and can be frustrating for women who experience this chronically, as evidenced by recurring yeast and bacterial infections (e.g. bacterial vaginosis) that respond to anti-fungals and antibiotics but keep coming back. I find that more often a woman will have an ongoing bad odor and/or more discharge than is normal, but it's never severe enough for her to seek out treatment. **Imbalances can modify pH and may slow the elimination of HPV.** An August 2014 review of literature that included 63 studies found a consistent correlation between bacterial imbalances of the vagina and persistent HPV [118]. HPV seems to be associated with a reduction in lactobacilli and an increase in the diversity of vaginal microbiota [48,49,50]. I must admit that I often see dysbioses in women who are slower to eliminate CIN and HPV regardless of the CIN severity. In these cases I may use essential oil suppositories to suppress unwanted bacteria and yeast and/or *Lactobacillus acidophilus* suppositories. Lactobacilli are the dominant microbiota in a healthy vaginal environment and help to suppress unhealthy bacteria by keeping the vagina slightly acidic. **A failure to address imbalances in vaginal microbiota may result in recalcitrant dysplasia, persistent HPV and disease recurrence.**

The correlation between bacteria and HPV persistence is not only limited to the vagina; research has identified a link between gingivitis and bacterial vaginosis (BV) [51]. Gingivitis is linked to BV, and BV is increases the likelihood of persistent HPV; therefore, it would seem reasonable to think that gingivitis increases HPV persistence. Given this potential relationship, it is wise to address oral health as part of a CIN/HPV treatment program. In other words, brush twice per day, floss at least once and if you have gingivitis get treatment. The practice of "oil pulling", the forceful swishing of coconut oil around your teeth for ten minutes, is a good habit to prevent gingivitis and maintain healthy populations of oral bacteria.

Because of research published in 2014, I have just begun using vitamin D suppositories in some of my cases (January 2015)*. This new addition to my practice is because the authors of this study found that after six weeks of vitamin D vaginal suppositories, used three nights per week, that there was "good anti-dysplastic effects" for CIN1 [119]. The results were not so good for CIN2, but as an added benefit 79% of the women in the study had "less vaginal problems", "less discharge" and "less problems with sexual intercourse." After 6 weeks of treatment only 7% of the patients still had bacterial and/or fungal vaginal infections that required treatment (to clarify, the study examined CIN1, CIN2 *and* chronic recurrent cervical infections/cervicitis).

Note: As of writing this vitamin D suppositories are not available; I had to have them custom-made. And I don't recommend using an oral vitamin D pill in this capacity(I say this to be pre-emptive: I have seen no small number of women put all sorts of things up there with the hope of getting rid of HPV—and sometimes to their detriment).

Common Questions:

1) **"Can I engage in sexual relations while undergoing escharotic treatment?"**
In years past I didn't have any suggested restrictions on intercourse but my position has changed a bit in response to research. I do not recommend abstinence during escharotic treatment; however, because HPV is found in the semen of men, I recommend using a condom—at least during treatment. This is to avoid potential "bathing" of an already irritated and vulnerable cervix with HPV. Once your pap is normal and you are HPV negative, your preferred method of contraception is up to you.

2) **"Can the virus be passed back and forth between partners?"**
I don't think so. Once you clear whatever strain(s) you have, it is unlikely that you can be re-infected with the same strain(s). I base this on a couple of observations: one, I don't think that I've ever had to re-treat a person for HPV, except when the patient has had additional new partners and likely was infected with a new strain of HPV (this is over the course of twenty years of treating HPV); two, the goal of treatment is for your immune system to recognize whatever strains that you have. Once this recognition is made, your immune system will prevent a re-infection with the same strain. For example, you can't get measles twice; once you are infected you will have permanent immunity against measles (this is different than with vaccination where the vaccine will not confer permanent immunity and you can get it later in life). Additionally, the chances are that at some point your partner will clear the virus as well, so there will be nothing to pass back and forth.

3)   "Can you get rid of HPV completely?"

I think so; at least I don't have any good reason to think not. There are very few viral infections that are permanent. Herpes virus is one, but that is because it "hides out" in the nervous system making it impossible for the immune system to attack it. Although HPV is pretty good at hiding as well, a person's immune system will find it under the right circumstances as evidenced by research demonstrating HPV16-specific cd4 cells in women who easily clear the virus [6]. Some conventional doctors claim that you can never get rid of HPV, but these opinions are coming from providers whose treatment ignores the virus, opting instead for the cutting out of diseased tissue.

4)   "Why hasn't my doctor recommended escharotic therapy if it's so effective?"

If you are still asking this question then you've missed the point of this book; I suggest reading it again, paying specific attention to what I've written about standard-of-care and the FDA in Chapter 3.

5)   "Will HPV or dysplasia come back after it is gone?"

I doesn't seem to, and of the very few women in which I've re-treated, there is good reason to think that they had a new strain of HPV (i.e. they had additional partners since their normal post-treatment pap). Furthermore, I've never had to re-treat a woman who maintained—and whose partner maintained--a monogamous relationship. Also, once your pap is normal and the virus is absent, I recommend taking a good multivitamin that contains methyl folate...*forever*. Studies have demonstrated that folic acid can prevent HPV infection, prevent dysplasia from worsening and help get rid of it entirely. It should also have an appreciable amount of vitamin D (at least 1000 IU) or you should take vitamin D as a separate supplement.

6)   "Should I be worried about anal HPV and anal dysplasia?"

At this point in time, there are no guidelines regarding who should test for anal HPV and when, although guidelines are certain to be forthcoming. If you have anal sex you should be tested for HPV (there is an anal "pap" that your doctor can perform). Also, if you are worried that you may have it then you should be tested. If anal HPV is present, I recommend seeing a proctologist or gastroenterologist to be screened for anal/rectal dysplasia. Better yet, don't have anal sex unless you are in a committed relationship with enough history to know that neither of you have HPV.

7)   "Should I be concerned about oral HPV?"

Absolutely. Most women who I see with genital HPV and CIN believe it to be one of the worst things ever. It is common for a patient to break down in tears and exclaim that she is never going to have sex again; however, oral, throat and lung HPV is worse—allow me to explain: women are regularly screened for HPV and CIN. If you find it, you can treat it and have no problems. But we don't routinely screen for oral HPV—at least not currently, because there are yet to be guidelines. This means that a person could fly under the radar for years and develop oral, throat or lung cancer. Screening guidelines are coming, but in the meantime I recommend that you have an oral HPV test if you are concerned. Any physician can order the oral HPV kits from their lab (I use Quest Diagnostics). Additionally, it seems prudent to refrain from oral sex with anyone except if in a committed long-term relationship where you are both HPV negative.

8)   **"Can men be tested for HPV?"**
Not yet, but probably soon. There is a urine test that should be on the market in 2015; although the thinking is that this will be another way to screen women, it will also be a way to screen men. Researchers and physicians are not concerned about testing men because there is no medical treatment for HPV. The associated thinking is "who cares if you have it because there is nothing that you can do about it". Although after reading this book you should recognize their error, they continue to make false claims and tell women "don't worry about HPV, you'll probably clear it and everybody has it". The value in screening men for HPV is that when you meet a prospective sex partner you can both be tested and make a decision how to move forward.
Note: As of April 2015 this test is not yet FDA-approved, but it is available at www.trovagene.com.

9)   **"Are men carriers of HPV?"**
Yes, men are carriers; and so are women. Every man walking around with HPV was infected by a woman (assuming heterosexuality). I make this point because I've treated women who were angry, blaming men as the source of their problem. Granted, infidelity may have caused an HPV infection and thus feelings of betrayal and anger, but without concrete knowledge of cheating, it is very difficult to determine *when* you were infected. Although it is my position that it is possible to eliminate HPV completely, there may be some of us who maintain infected cells without active viral replication, showing negative on testing despite being infected. Because of this, my recommendation is forget about trying to determine *when* you were infected; it doesn't matter. All that matters is getting rid of CIN and testing negative for the virus.

10)   **"Do condoms prevent HPV transmission?"**
Short answer: no. Long answer: maybe a little bit but for all intents and purposes, do not rely on condoms to prevent HPV transmission. A condom will do nothing at all to prevent wart strains of HPV (we don't generally test

for wart strains, of which there are dozens, because they don't tend to cause cancer). This is because virus is all over the genital area and a condom only covers the penis, not the surrounding skin that is making contact with you. This is the same reason why many people get herpes while using condoms. High-risk HPV is more likely to be found in the semen, which is why I said that condoms may protect "a little bit", at least from the high-risk viruses (these we do test for routinely and there are 13-14 strains at this point in time). Bottom line advice: have prospective partners, and yourself, get tested before sexual relations. This practice may put a damper on your Saturday night, but it's better than getting a raging herpetic outbreak a week later or CIN3 one to two years later.

11) **"Is HPV a sexually transmitted disease?"**

Yes and no. HPV can certainly be transmitted by sexual activities, but there are other ways to contract the virus. Many infants are born with it—gotten through vaginal delivery or while developing as a fetus (HPV has been identified in amniotic fluid). There is a good chance that if you walk on the floors of public bathrooms/showers barefoot you have been exposed to it. In effect, *any* wart on your body is HPV. You can auto-infect, or *auto-inoculate*, as well; in other words, if you have a genital infection you may be able to spread it to your face or elsewhere via your own fingers. It can be spread female to female as well as male to male. It can also be spread via sex toys or any inanimate objects (it can survive on the surfaces of things for about 1 week). It may be spread with open-mouthed kissing as well. My advice: rather than freak out knowing that the virus may be all over the place, exercise good judgment in choosing sex partners and most importantly, *take care of yourself*! As you've discovered in this book, you can help to prevent HPV infections as well as decrease the likelihood that the virus will cause problems by eating well and taking nutritional supplements. In fact, this is precisely what I recommend to my patients after the completion of treatment: continue eating a lot of greens, vegetables and fruits—also take a good multivitamin with methyl folate and phytochemicals *forever.*

12) **"Can escharotic solutions be used for external warts?"**

No. External warts are best treated with either freezing or Aldara® (imiquimod) cream. I use freezing for solitary lesions and recommend the cream if there are numerous warts over a large area. The cream actually works very well so I do not recommend messing around with alternative treatments for something that responds so well to conventional treatment. Internal vaginal warts are an exception; escharotic treatments will eliminate them.

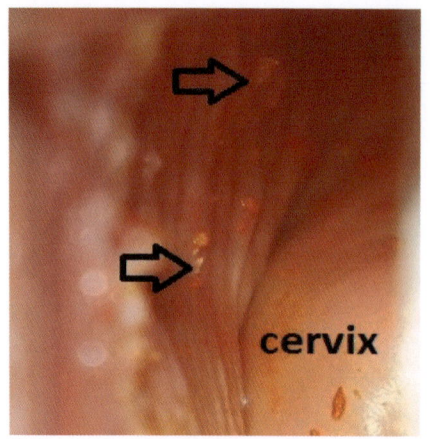 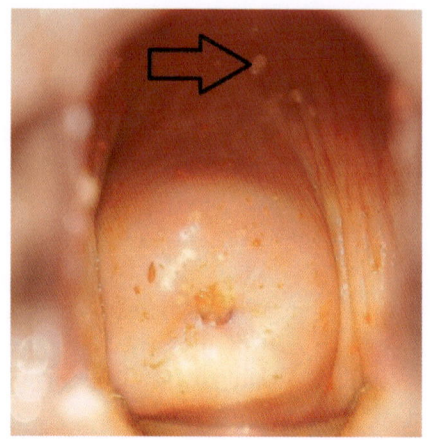

These are the images of the cervix and vaginal walls of a 32-year old woman after the initial escharotic application for persistent HPV, genital warts and cervical dysplasia. She had a LEEP performed 6 months prior for CIN2/3 but the dysplasia had returned. Additionally, she was struggling with foot, hand and genital warts for over two years. The arrows in the images above show internal warts on the vaginal walls. *Note that some orange-colored bumps are debris, not warts which are pointy in appearance.*

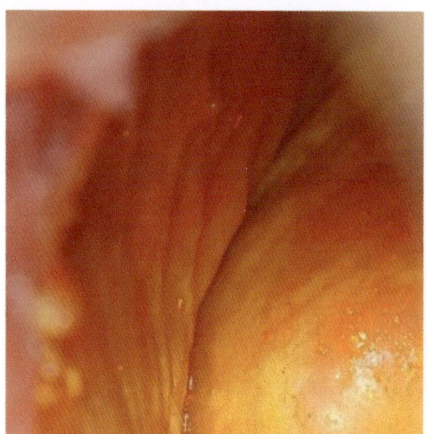 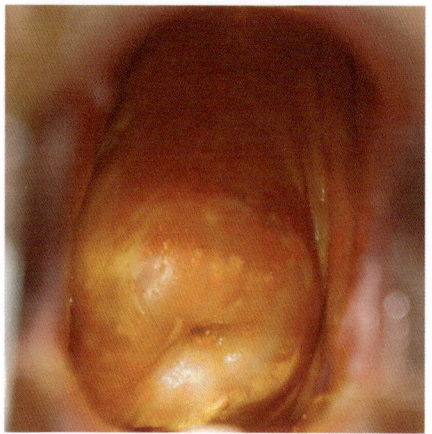

These images were taken 1 week later. The internal warts which were clearly visible at the time of the initial treatment are now gone. With this second application there are areas of staining that were not evident with the first application; this is typical and represents either HPV-infected cells that are not dysplastic or areas of inflammation. After treatment her pap was normal, HPV negative and the external warts were eliminated with Aldara®.

13) **"Is the treatment painful"**

About 50% of the time there will be some discomfort. When it does occur, it usually consists of mild cramping but can be severe in about 5-10% of patients. However, I've never had a case that was so painful that treatment had to be discontinued.

14) **"How effective is the treatment?"**

It is very effective. Nearly every case of cervical dysplasia that I've treated since 1995 has been eliminated; however, my high success rate is likely due to the fact that I treat until it is gone, whether it takes 8 treatments or 28 treatments. Fortunately, the average number of escharotic applications to eliminate CIN is 8-12, regardless of whether it is mild or severe. The success rate of testing negative for HPV is about 90% by the end of treatment for premenopausal women and about 70% for those who are post-menopausal. I believe that this disparity that is age-dependent is due to the fact that as we age our immune system function diminishes, making it more difficult to clear the virus. If the virus is not cleared by the time the CIN is gone, I usually recommend continuing to work at getting rid of it by maintaining a healthy diet and by taking most of the supplements that I recommend for treatment. Most women will go on to clear the virus within a year—and these are women who have had persistent infections and a protracted history of cervical abnormalities and surgical interventions.

15) **"Should I get the HPV vaccine?"**

As of April 2015, I cannot recommend HPV vaccines. Both the safety and effectiveness of the Gardasil® and Cervarix® vaccines remain uncertain. A serious discussion of this topic would be a book in itself, so I will stick to the main issues for the sake of brevity. The biggest problem with evaluating the effectiveness is that in "fast-tracking" the vaccines for approval, the FDA violated its own requirements and made potentially erroneous assumptions on insufficient data (only 3 years worth). In effect, it was assumed that any diminished dysplasia attributed to the vaccines was a prevention of cancer. However, dysplasia will often clear without any intervention making the assumption invalid. More recently, Drs. Lucija Tomljenovic and Chris Shaw, researchers from the University of British Columbia, have demonstrated that the vaccines have not prevented any cancer whatsoever, nor are they likely to—at least not in developed countries with robust cervical screening programs. Because it can take many years for cervical cancer to develop, it will be decades before we have enough data to determine whether they actually work. However, if effectiveness was my only concern, I would probably recommend inoculation with the vaccine in the hope that it *might* work. **The problem is, however, that there have been a disproportionate number of adverse events associated with Gardasil® and Cervarix®.** From 2006 to 2013, the Vaccine Adverse Event Reporting System (VAERS) reported over 26,000 adverse events for HPV vaccines, 92 deaths, 866 cases of permanent disability and over 9,000 injuries requiring emergency hospitalization. VAERS is the United States Health and Human Services vaccine injury reporting agency. Of significant concern is the fact that HPV vaccines account for over 60% of *all* reported vaccine injuries. Concerns over safety have led the Japanese Health Ministry to withdraw its recommendation to vaccinate for HPV and other countries are investigating their safety and efficacy as well. Because there is so much money to be made by U.S. pharma companies producing vaccines, it's challenging to get accurate information. Furthermore, in the U.S., vaccine manufacturers cannot be sued for vaccine injuries, which results in a lack of transparency that benefits manufacturers while putting the public at risk. **At this point in time, it appears that HPV vaccines have more risk than benefit.**

16) **"How do I find a practitioner who provides escharotic therapy?"**
Finding a practitioner can be challenging. The most likely escharotic practitioners are chiropractors and naturopaths. Most states do not license naturopaths and thus they cannot perform the treatment and although chiropractors are licensed in every state, some states restrict their scope of practice and thus they cannot perform escharotic therapy. As a result, there are probably only about thirteen or fourteen states where you may find a practitioner. Additionally, even in states where it can be done, you are not likely going to find a provider that has sufficient experience. I do not know of anyone outside of the U.S. providing this therapy; however, it is my goal to change that by providing training at my clinic in Chicago. My recommendation is to do an internet search for escharotic therapy in your geographic location.

17) **"Is escharotic treatment the same as Black Salve treatment?"**
A "Black Salve" is an externally-applied ointment or paste that typically contains bloodroot, varying concentrations of zinc chloride and other substances, purported to treat a wide variety of cancers. Although similar to the escharotic used in my natural treatment, there are fundamental differences that cast doubt on the alleged success of these salves. One, the bloodroot has no way to make direct contact with the abnormal cell because the skin forms an effective barrier; thus, the *sanguinarine* cannot shut down sodium-potassium pumps. This is in contrast to the cervix where it can be applied *directly* to the abnormal cells, killing them as a result. Two, the protocol for using most salves is to apply it to the area overlying the suspected tumor and to leave it *for days*. This allows the zinc chloride to eventually "eat" a hole through the skin. When an escharotic solution is applied to the cervix, it is left for 90 seconds *and then removed,* thereby minimizing damage to any normal tissue in the vicinity. Recently, I

performed a breast thermogram on a woman who had used a Black Salve for her breast cancer. The salve destroyed the better part of her breast, leaving a ghastly wound that would not heal. Not only did the salve not get rid of the cancer, it delayed what would have likely been more appropriate care, and she had to have surgery anyway. **Black Salves can be dangerous. I do not recommend their use for anything.** They are completely different than the escharotic therapy for cervical dysplasia that I've described in this book.

18)   Can I do treatment on myself?

No, the treatment solution can be hazardous if used improperly and putting the solution on the cervix requires looking at it with the aid of a speculum. All in all this would be extremely difficult and unwise to attempt. *I actually added this question as I was about to send the manuscript to the publisher because someone actually asked me if she could do treatment on herself.*

19)   "Are there any side effects or scarring of the cervix?"

Not only is there never scarring caused by escharotic treatment, it actually can eliminate cervicitis and scarring/mutilation caused by previous LEEPs and cones. In this regard it appears to act as a chemical peel, facilitating the growth of healthy tissue.

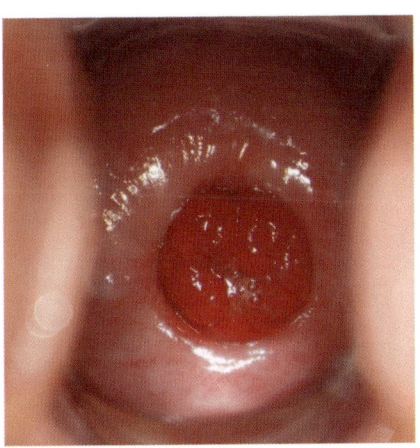 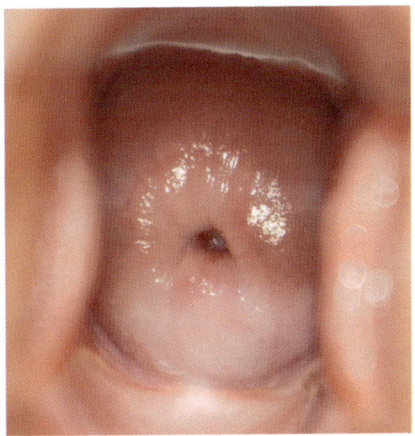

The image on the left is the cervix of a 26-year old woman at the beginning of treatment for CIN2. She had a LEEP performed seven years prior that has disfigured her cervix (the red area). The image on the right is her cervix after eight applications of escharotic solution. Although this appears to be a dramatic transformation of a damaged cervix, improvements such as this are the rule, not the exception.

Chapter 5-HPV and Cervical Dysplasia Case Studies

Case 1: Normal pap, High-risk HPV+

Kim was a 42-year old who had known that she was HR-HPV positive for at least three years prior to seeing me. Although a pap smear performed 6 months prior to her initial visit with me was LSIL (probably mild dysplasia), the most recent pap taken several months before her first visit was normal. Kim was an otherwise healthy woman without any other significant health concerns.

The treatment that I recommend for women with normal pap smears but who are HPV+ is very similar to the treatment for dysplasia—escharotic applications, supplements and dietary changes. Because Kim resided in Chicago, we did weekly escharotic applications and I put her on a multi-vitamin, DIM, methyl folate, vitamin D, a mushroom extract, curcumin and a bacillus probiotic. I also had her taking 2,000mg of vitamin C and monolauric acid to improve her immunity.

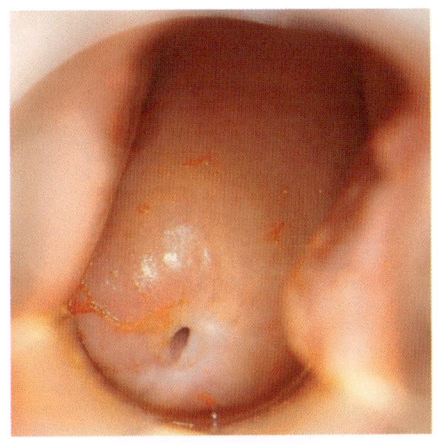

Image 1: After the initial application of the escharotic solution, there isn't any appreciable staining of abnormal cells; this is expected considering that her pap was normal. Typically, the more abnormal the cell, the faster the staining occurs. I find that with HPV alone, more staining will occur on the second or third applications.

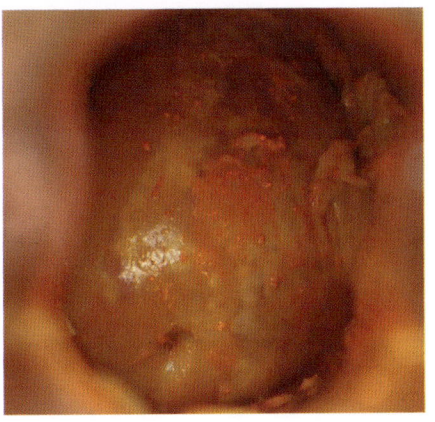

Image 2: Note that at the time of the second treatment there are areas that are staining (the white areas). Because curcumin was added with this treatment, everything appears yellow/orange. There are also areas in which a thin layer of dead cells is peeling off.

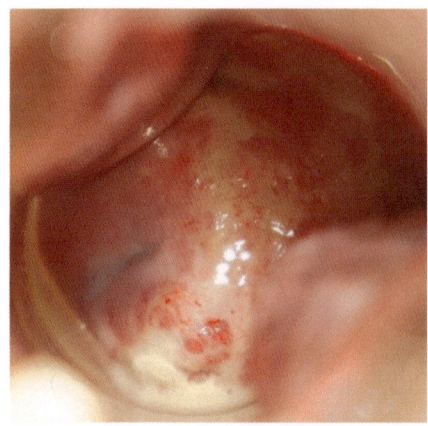

Image 3: After two treatments, areas of HPV infection are dying (the white area). Note that this image is before the escharotic is applied for the third time.

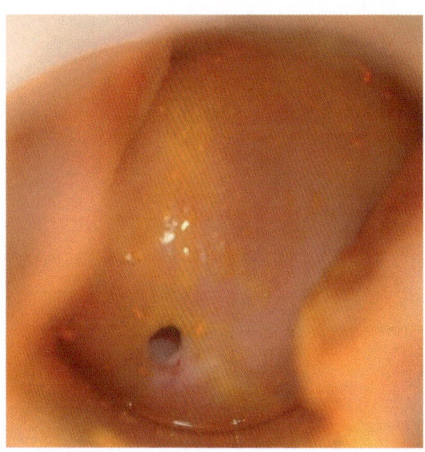

Image 4: This is the image of Kim's cervix after the seventh and final treatment. There isn't any staining occurring, indicating that all HPV-infected cells should have been eliminated. Kim's 6-week follow-up pap smear was HPV negative, as were her 3-month and 6-month tests.

Case 2: CIN3 ectocervix, CIN3 canal, HR-HPV+

Marcy was a 48-year old perimenopausal woman who was positive for high-risk HPV and had CIN3 on the outer cervix as well as CIN3 in the endocervical canal. Interestingly enough, this was her first abnormal pap smear ever. Marcy was an otherwise healthy, successful woman.

The treatment that we began was my standard oral supplements, a plant-based diet and escharotic applications. Because Marcy was flying to Chicago, we did two consecutive treatments about three weeks apart--as opposed to weekly applications--to minimize the cost of travel.

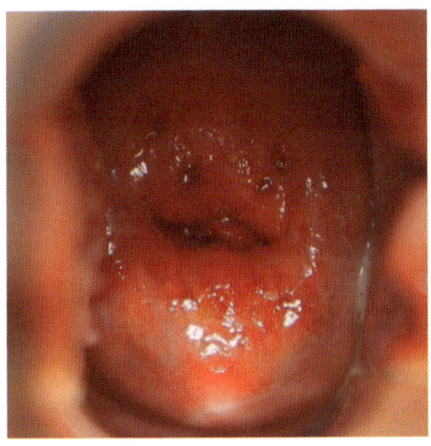

Image 1: Marcy's cervix was not healthy; she had cervicitis as indicated by the redness, inflammation and Nabothian cysts (the dark red spots which are actually pits where the cysts have ruptured). Also, there is a polyp, a benign tumor that usually will protrude from the opening (it appears like a tiny red tongue poking out of the canal). Often, polyps will be a source of spotting in older women. This image was taken before any treatment was started.

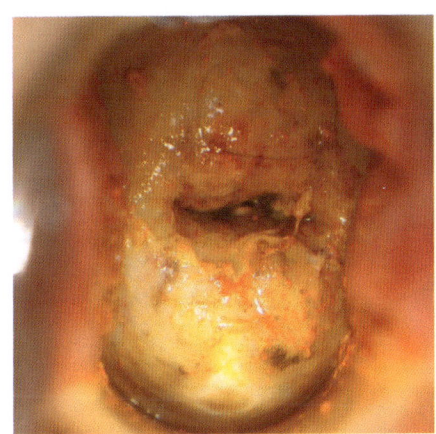

Image 2: This image was after 3 treatments. The entire cervix has been affected by the escharotic and the surface is sloughing off. Although this is a large area that is involved, it is not all dysplasia; cells that are inflamed will also stain and die with treatment.

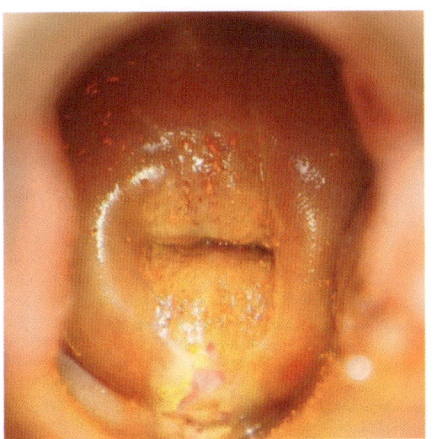

Image 3: After five escharotic applications the majority of the inflammation is gone and the area that is staining is much smaller. However, because there continues to be staining around the canal opening, treatment will continue.

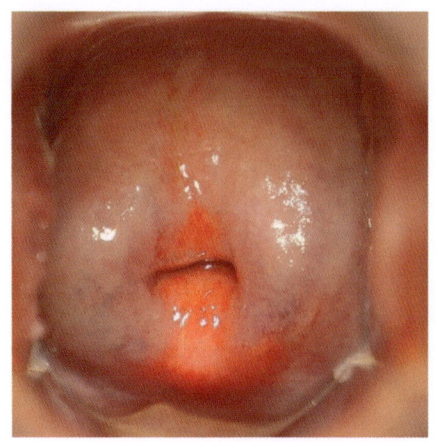

Image 4: After 11 treatments, Marcy's cervix is looking much healthier. Most of the inflammation and the Nabothian cysts are gone. This image was taken before applying the final escharotic solution. Observe that the polyp is also gone. In addition to being highly effective at eliminating abnormal cells, the escharotic acts like a chemical peel, facilitating the resurfacing of what had been an unhealthy cervix.

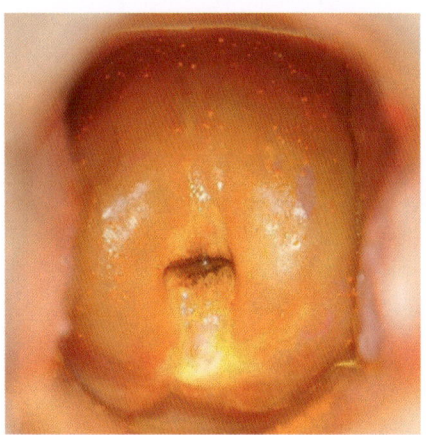

Image 5: This image was taken after applying the escharotic on the same day as image 4. Although there continues to be staining—mostly above and below the canal—I decided to discontinue treatment because I suspected that the little bit of staining that remained was due to inflammation rather than dysplasia. Marcy had a pap done 6 weeks later that was normal with negative HPV.

Case 3: Cervical CIN2; HR-HPV+; History of vaginal and cervical cancer

Amy, a 51-year old perimenopausal woman, had a history of cervical and vaginal cancer—both of which were localized (*in situ*). Amy had surgery to remove both cancers but within one year CIN2 was identified on her cervix. Surgery was again recommended but she had lost confidence in her doctors and in the conventional approach to HPV; she was desperate for an alternative.

Just like the patient in the previous case, Amy was flying in to Chicago for treatment so we did two days of consecutive treatment and repeated this once per month. Because Amy was having serious problems with the virus (she had already had both vaginal and cervical cancer) my oral treatment regimen was aggressive, using all supplements with evidentiary support. This is in contrast to women with recent dysplasia, especially if mild, where the need for aggressive treatment has less justification.

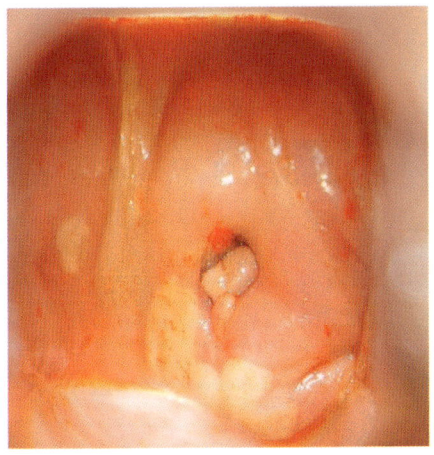

Image 1: This image was taken after the first escharotic application. The staining is localized to the lower cervix and a small area on the vaginal wall.

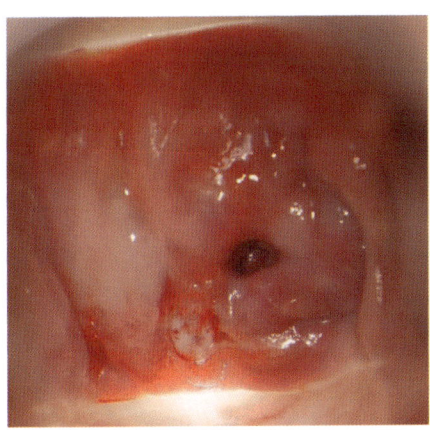

Image 2: After 4 treatments, this is the appearance of Amy's cervix. Note that there is redness and inflammation that correspond to the areas that were staining in image 1; this denotes areas of ongoing death of abnormal cells over the course of the last four treatments.

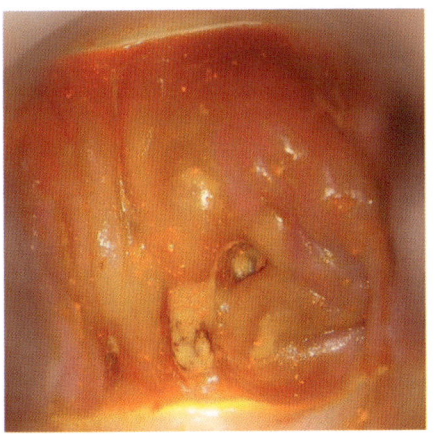

Image 3: This image was taken on the same day as image 2 after applying the escharotic. Note that the areas that are staining are a little smaller than at the time of the initial treatment in image 1.

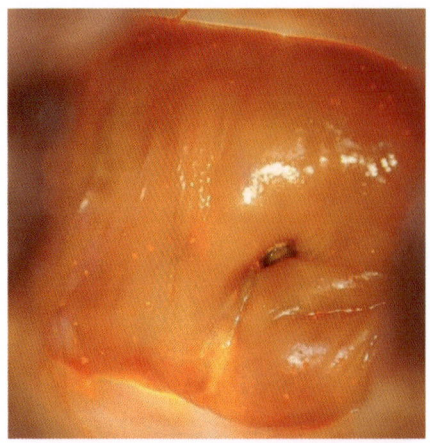

Image 4: Amy's cervix was looking much better after applying the ninth and final treatment. The very small area of staining below the opening was probably inflammation because it was still in the process of healing. Treatment was discontinued with the decision to perform a pap in 6 weeks. Doing a pap smear without enough time for the cervix to fully heal can result in an "ASCUS" pap smear; this is due to lingering inflammation.

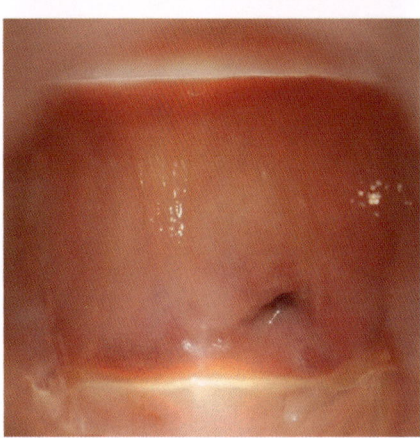

Image 5: This picture was taken at the time of Amy's pap smear. The cervix had healed very well. Her pap smear was normal and HPV was not detected. She continued with some of the supplements initially prescribed to minimize the likelihood of having future problems; this is especially important in women who've had persistent HPV or recurrent dysplasia.

Case 4: Cervical and endocervical CIN3 with HPV-16

Linda was a 23-year old who came to me a couple of months after a LEEP/conization for severe dysplasia. The surgical procedure had not gotten rid of all of the dysplasia and CIN3 was still in the canal and on the outer cervix. Her first abnormal pap smear with high-risk HPV occurred when she was 19; she was told at that time that she didn't need to do anything and the Gardasil vaccine was recommended.

Linda had been using a Mirena IUD for a couple of years. We decided to leave the IUD in place for the duration of treatment provided that she was responding well to treatment; in the event that she was responding slowly, we agreed to remove it.

Oral treatment consisted of DIM/I3C, a multi-vitamin, curcumin, methyl-folate and vitamin D. I also recommended that she increase her consumption of dark, leafy greens, yellow/orange vegetables and fruits. Escharotic therapy began at a frequency of once per week.

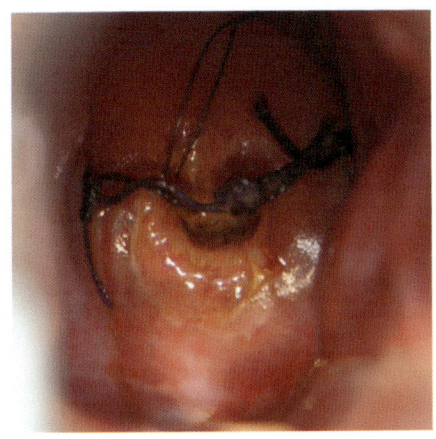

Image 1: This image is after the initial application of escharotic. Although CIN3 is present, the area of involvement is not large (the white/orange stained area). The dark string is suture stitching to close up the cervix after the conization procedure. The thinner string on the upper cervix is attached to the IUD to allow for its removal.

Image2: This image was taken after the 4th treatment. The area that is now staining is less than half of what it had been at start of therapy.

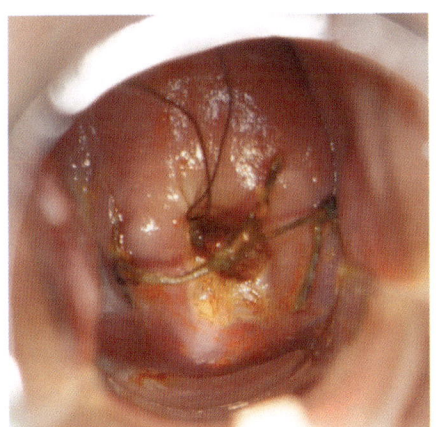

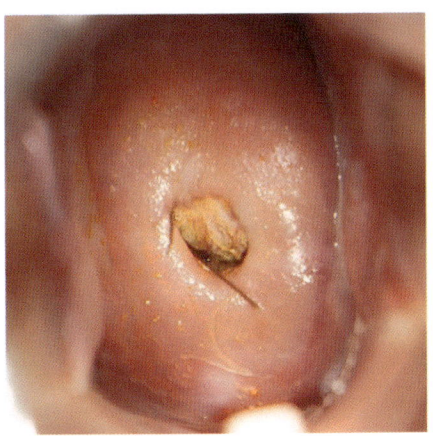

Image 3: Since the 4th treatment (image 2), the sutures had been removed. The cervix is looking much better but there is still staining just inside of the canal. This was the ninth treatment and we decided to remove the progestin-secreting IUD. As cervical cells become increasingly dysplastic, the number of progesterone receptors increase. To avoid stimulating these cells with the synthetic progesterone, we removed the IUD.

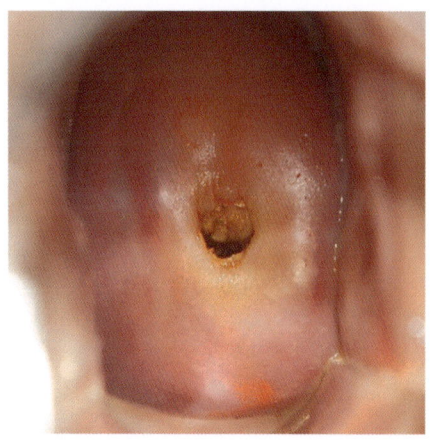

Image 4: This was after the 16th escharotic application. Because there is still some staining in the canal, we continued treatment.

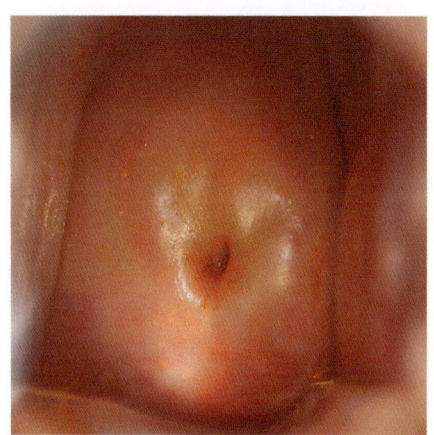

Image 4: This was after the 21st and final treatment. There is no longer staining and the cervix appears healthy. Linda's case was unusual because of the number of treatments required to eliminate the dysplasia. Most cases require 8-12 applications; however, in about 10% of women it can take over 15 treatments.

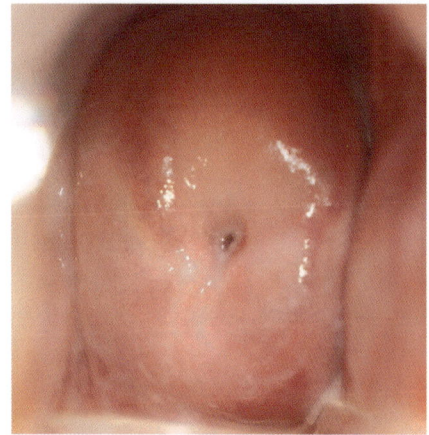

Image 5: This picture was taken at the time of Linda's pap smear. After struggling with HPV and dysplasia for almost 5 years, her pap smear was normal and HPV negative. In the three years since the conclusion of treatment, Linda's pap has remained normal and HPV negative.

Case 5: CIN1 with HPV-16; Cervicitis

Mary was a 32-year old woman with 2 children, CIN1 and HPV-16. She did not want to follow her doctor's advice to do no treatment and "watch and wait", repeating a pap smear every 6 months. She was in the middle of a divorce and felt that HPV would impair her ability to move on with her life. Additionally, she felt "diseased" and was struggling with the ethics of whether she would have to tell any future relationship prospects that she had HPV.

I often base the aggressiveness of oral therapy on the severity of dysplasia as well as the finances of the patient; I also base it on the degree to which a patient wants be aggressive. In other words, if a patient wants do to "everything under the sun" to eliminate HPV, I am more likely to prescribe additional supplements. With regard to Mary, she had mild dysplasia and the financial burden of kids and divorce, so I tried to keep the cost of treatment to a minimum. Her oral treatment consisted of a multi-vitamin, DIM/I3C and methyl folate.

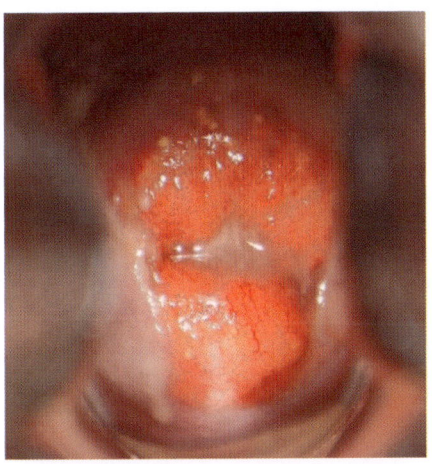

Image 1: This is Mary's cervix before we started therapy. In addition to CIN1, the presence of Nabothian cysts (yellow spots on upper cervix) and redness indicate cervicitis. Escharotic therapy was initiated at a frequency of once per week.

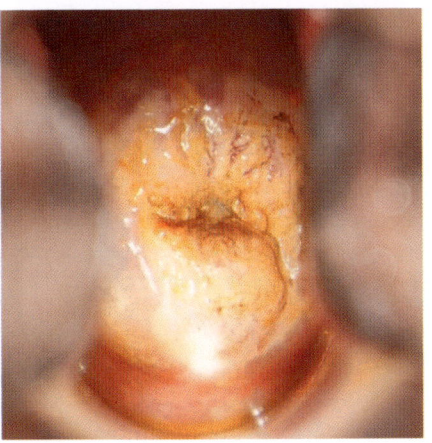

Image 2: This image was taken after the first application of bloodroot and ZnCl. The area that has stained (white/yellow) denotes both dysplasia and inflammation.

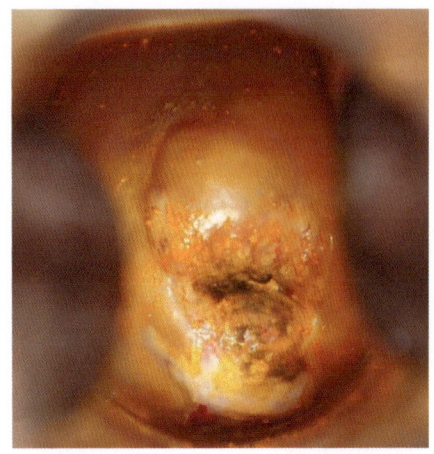

Image 3: This picture was taken immediately after the sixth escharotic application. The addition of curcumin to the treatment solution colors the entire cervix a yellow/orange color. Note that the area that was staining is much smaller than in image 2. Because everything was coming along as expected, nothing was altered with her treatment plan and we continued with weekly applications.

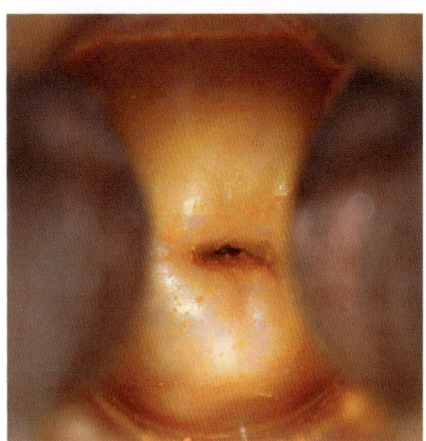

Image 5: This image was taken after the 11th escharotic application. There wasn't any staining and the decision was made to do a pap smear in 6 weeks. Marys' pap was normal and HPV negative.

Case 6: HSIL pap; normal biopsy; HR-HPV+

Diane was a 27-year old woman who had an abnormal pap smear seven years prior to seeing me. For the preceding four years, she had been having consistently abnormal pap smears but all colposcopic examinations had been normal. The last pap prior to seeking my care was HSIL, suggesting moderate to severe dysplasia, despite the colposcopic examination and biopsies being normal.

In Diane's case--as is common with all similar cases in which a pap smear is abnormal but colpos are normal—her doctor wanted to perform a conization, removing a large part of the cervical canal, believing that the persistent pap abnormality must be coming from an "undetected and unseen" lesion in the canal. This approach relies on guesswork as opposed to science. I have found in similar cases that the abnormalities usually originate on the vaginal walls and/or the area where the cervix attaches to the vaginal wall--not deep in the canal. I base this hypothesis on the fact that there is typically staining on the walls when I perform escharotic treatment and all similar cases that I have treated have always resolved when the vaginal walls are treated.

Diane's treatment consisted of the usual supplements that I prescribe, a plant-based diet and weekly escharotic applications.

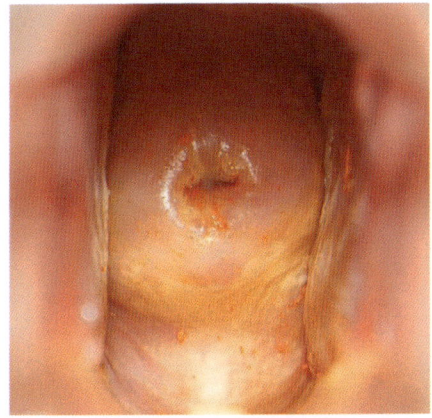

Image 1: This image was taken after the initial application of bloodroot and ZnCl. Note that although there was a little staining around the canal, perhaps due to some minor inflammation, the areas on the upper and lower cervix as well as the lateral vaginal walls close to the cervix are staining prominently (the white areas). For these areas to stain so quickly and prominently is suggestive of dysplasia as opposed to HVP-infected cells that are otherwise healthy.

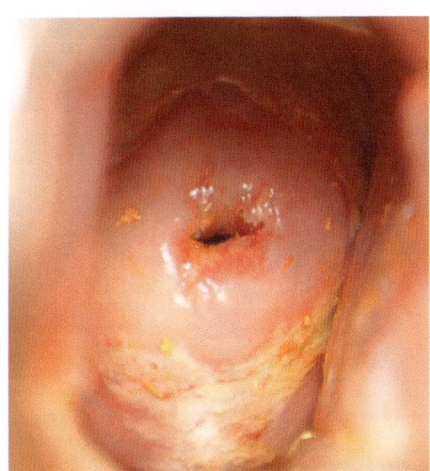

Image 2: In confirmation of my suspicions as outlined in Image 1, eschars (scab-like formations) have formed in the areas that were staining at the time of the first application. This picture was taken after the second escharotic application.

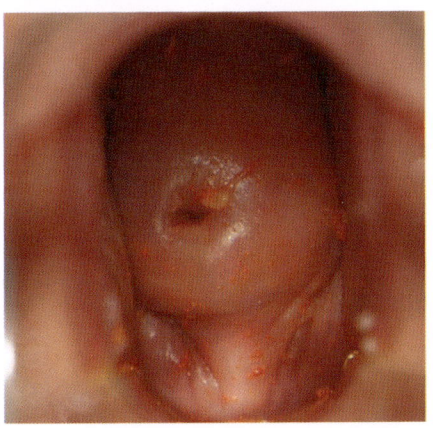

Image 3: This is a picture taken after the 8th and final escharotic application. There is no longer any staining visible on the cervix, the vaginal walls or any areas in between. A pap smear was performed 6 weeks later that was normal and HPV negative. This was Diane's first normal pap smear in over four years.

References

1. Nelson EL, Stockdale CK. 2013. Vulvar and vaginal HPV disease. Obstet Gynecol Clin N Am. 40:359-376.

2. Doerfler D, Bernhaus A, et al. 2009. Human papilloma virus infection prior to coitarche. Am J Obstet Gynecol. May;200(5).

3. World Health Organization-International Agency for Research on Cancer. An introduction to cervical intraepithelial neoplasia (CIN). Available from http://www.screening.iarc.fr/colpochap.php?chap=2.

4. Longworth, Laimins M, Laimins L. 2004. Pathogenesis of Human Papillomaviruses in Differentiating Epithelia. 68,no.2:362-372. Accessed 9 Mar 2014. doi:10.1128/MMBR.68.2362-372.2004.E

5. Meyer SI, Fuglsang K, Blaakaer J. 2014. Cell-mediated immune response: a clinical review of the therapeutic potential of human papillomavirus vaccination. Acta Obstet Gynecol Scand. Dec;93(12):1209-18. doi: 10.1111/aogs.12480.Epub 2014 Sep 20.

6. Peng S, Trimble C, Wu L, et al. 2007. HLA-DQB1*02-restricted HPV-16 E7 peptide-specific CD4 T-cell immune responses correlate with regression of HPV-16-associated high-grade squamous intraepithelial lesions. Clinical Cancer Research: an official journal of the American Association for Cancer Research. 13(8):2479-2487. doi:10.1158/1078-0432.CCR-06-2916.

7. Williams VM, Filippova M, Filippov V, Payne KJ, Duerksen-Hughes P. 2014. Human papillomavirus type 16 E6* induces oxidative stress and DNA damage. J Virol. Jun;88(12):6751-61. doi: 10.1128/JVI.03355-13. Epub 2014 Apr 2.

8. Giampieri S, Storey A. 2004. Repair of UV-induced thymine dimmers is compromised in cells expressing the E6 protein from human papillomaviruses types 5 and 18. Br J Cancer. 90:2203-2209.

9. Mazurek S, Zwerschke W, Jansen-Durr P, Eigenbrodt E. 2001. Effects of the human papilloma virus HPV-16 E7 oncoprotein on glycolysis and glutaminolysis: Role of pyruvate kinase type M2 and the glycolytic-enzyme complex. Biochem J. 356:247-256. doi: 10.1042/0264-6021:3560247.

10. Zhang E, Feng X, Liu F, Zhang P, Liang J, Tang X. 2014. Roles of PI3K/Akt and c-Jun signaling pathways in human papillomavirus type 16 oncoprotein-induced HIF-1α, VEGF, and IL-8 expression and in vitro angiogenesis in non-small cell lung cancer cells. PLos One. Jul 24;9(7):e103440. doi: 10.1371/journal.pone.0103440.ecollection.

11. Paavonen J, Koutsky LA, Kaviat N. 1990. Cervical neoplasia and other STD-related genital and anal neoplasias. In: KK Holmes, PA Mardh, PG Sparling, PJ Wiegener (eds.) Sexually Transmitted Diseases. New York: McGraw-Hill. P. 561-592.

12.   Arbeit JM, Howley PM, Hanahan D. 1996. Chronic estrogen-induced cervical and vaginal squamous carcinogenesis in human papillomavirus type 16 transgenic mice. Proc Natl Acad Sci. 93:2930-2935.

13.   Crews MG, Taper LJ, Ritchey SJ. 1980. Effects of oral contraceptive agents on copper and zinc balance in young women. Am J Clin Nutr, 33:1940-1945.

14.   Daura-Oller E, Cabre M, Montero MA, Patemain JL, Romeu A. 2009. Specific gene hypomethylation and cancer: New insights into coding region feature trends. Bioinformation, 3(8): 340-343. doi: 10 6026/9732 0630003340.

15.   Cohen N, Kenigsberg E, Tanay A. 2011. Primate CpG islands are maintained by heterogeneous evolutionary regimes involving minimal selection". Cell 145 (5): 773–786.doi:10.1016/j.cell.2011.04.024. PMID 21620139.

16.   Piyathilake CJ, Henao OL, Macaluso M, et al. 2004. Folate is associated with the natural history of high-risk human papillomaviruses. Cancer Res.64(23):8788-8793.

17.   Piyathilake CJ, Macaluso M, Brill I, et al. 2007. Lower red blood cell folate enhances the HPV-16-associated risk of cervical intraepithelial neoplasia. Nutrition. 23(3): 203-210.

18.   Weinstein SJ, Ziegler RG, Rongillo EA, et al. 2001. Low serum and red blood cell folate are moderately, but not significantly associated with increased risk of invasive cervical cancer in US women. J Nutr. 131:2040-2048.

19.   Ziegler RG, Weinstein SJ, Fears TR. 2002. Nutritional and genetic inefficiencies in one-carbon metabolism and cervical cancer risk. J Nutr. 132:2345-2349.

20.   Thompson SW, Heimburger DC, Cornwell PE, et al. 2000. Effects of total plasma homocysteine on cervical dysplasia risk. Nutr Cancer. 37:128-133.

21.   Yu L, Chang K, Han J, Deng S, Chen M. 2013. Association between Methylenetetrahydrofolate reductase C677T polymorphism and susceptibility to cervical cancer: A meta-analysis. PLoS One,vol.8, issue 2, e55835.

22.   Xiong YH, He L, Fei J. 2014. Genetic variations in cytotoxic T-lymphocyte antigen-4 and susceptibility to cervical cancer. Int Immunopharmacol. 18(1):71-6. doi: 10.1016/j.intimp.2013.10.018. Epub 2013 Nov 4.

23.   Xia L, Gao J, Liu Y, Wu K. 2013. Significant association between CYP1A1 T3801C polymorphism and cervical neoplasia risk: as systemic review and meta-analysis. Tumour Biol. 34(1):223-30. doi: 10.1007/s13277-012-0542-9. Epub 2012 Oct 4.

24.   Tong SY, Lee JM, Song ES, Lee KB, et al. 2009. Functional polymorphism in manganese superoxide dismutase and antioxidant status: their interactions on the risk of cervical intraepithelial neoplasia and cervical cancer. Gynecol Oncol. 115(2):272-6. doi: 10.1016/j.ygyno.2009.07.032. Epub 2009 Aug 25.

25.   Sui Y, Han W, Yang Z, Jiang M, Li J. 2011. Association of glutathione S-transferase M1 and T1 null polymorphisms with the development of cervical lesions: a meta-analysis. Eur J Gynecol Reprod Biol. 159(2):443-8. doi: 10.1016/j.ejogrb.2011.09.012. Epub 2011 Oct 2.

26.   Zhen S, Hu CM, Bian LH. 2013. Glutathione S-transferase polymorphism interactions with smoking status and HPV infection in cervical cancer risk: an evidence-based meta-analysis. PLoS One. 8(12):e83497. doi: 10.1371/journal.pone.0083497. eCollection 2013.

27.   Moktar A, Singh R, Vadhanam MV, Ravoori S, Lillard JW, Gairola CG, Gupta RC. 2011. Cigarette smoke condensate-induced oxidative DNA damage and its removal in human cervical cancer cells. Int J Oncol. 39(4):941-7. doi: 10.3892/ijo.2011.1106. Epub 2011 Jun 29.

28.   Wei L, Griego AM, Chu M, Ozbun MA. 2014. Tobacco exposure results in increased E6 and E7 oncogene expression, DNA damage and mutation rates in cells maintaining episomal human papillomavirus 16 genomes. Carcinogenesis. Jul 26. pii: bgu156.

29.   Marszall M, Czarnowski W. 2007. Smoking influence on the level of homocysteine and 5-methyltetrahydrofolic acid in active and non smokers. Przegl Lek. 64(10):685-8.

30.   Scheurer ME, Danysh HE, Follen M, Lupo PJ. 2014. Association of traffic-related hazardous air pollutants and cervical dysplasia in an urban multiethnic population: a cross-sectional study. Environ Health. 13(1):52. doi: 10.1186/1476-069X-13-52.

31.   Munoz N, Franseschi S, Bosetti C, et al. 2002. Role of parity and human papillomavirus in cervical cancer: the IARC multicentric case-control study. Lancet. 30;359(9312):1093-101.

32.   Jensen KE, Schmiedel S, Norrild B et al. 2013. Parity as a cofactor for high-grade cervical disease among women with persistent human papillomavirus infection: a 13-year follow-up. Br J Cancer. 15;108(1):234-9. doi: 10.1038/bjc.2012.513. Epub 2012 Nov 20.

33.   International Collaboration of Epidemiological Studies of Cervical Cancer, Appleby P, Beral V, Berrington De Gonzalez A, et al. 2007. Cervical cancer and hormonal contraceptives: collaborative reanalysis of individual data for 16,573 women with cervical cancer and 35,509 women without cervical cancer from 24 epidemiological studies. Lancet. 10;370(9599):1609-21.

34.   Chih HJ, Lee AH, Colville L, Xu D, Binns CW. 2014. Condom and oral contraceptive use and risk of cervical intraepithelial neoplasia in

Australian women. J Gynecol Oncol. 25(3):183-7. doi: 10.3802/jgo.2014.25.3.183. Epub 2014 Jul 3.

35.	La Vecchia C, Boccia S. 2014. Oral contraceptives, human papillomavirus and cervical cancer. Eur J Cancer Prev. 23(2):110-2. doi: 10.1097/CEJ.0000000000000000.

36.	Amaral CM, Cetkovska K, Gurgel AP, Cardoso MV, et al. 2014. MDM2 polymorphism associated with the development of cervical lesions in women infected with human papillomavirus and using of oral contraceptives. Infect Agent Cancer. 18;9:24. doi: 10.1186/1750-9378-9-24. eCollection 2014.

37.	Chagas BS, Gurgel AP, da Cruz HL, et al. 2013. An interleukin-10 gene polymorphism associated with the development of cervical lesions in women infected with human papillomavirus and using oral contraceptives. Infect Genet Evol. 19:32-7. doi: 10.1016/j.meegid.2013.06.016. Epub 2013 Jun 22.

38.	Castellsague X, Diaz M, Vaccarella S, et al. 2011. Intrauterine device use, cervical infection with human papillomavirus, and risk of cervical cancer: a pooled analysis of 26 epidemiological studies. Lancet Oncol. 12(11):1023-31. doi: 10.1016/S1470-2045(11)70223-6. Epub 2011 Sep 12.

39.	Nikolaou M, Koumoundourou D, Ravazoula P, et al. 2014. An immunohistochemical analysis of sex-steroid receptors, tumor suppressor gene p53 and Ki-67 in the normal and neoplastic uterine cervix squamous epithelium. Med Pregl. 67(7-8):202-7.

40.	Cho H, Kim MK, Lee JK, et al. 2009. Relationship of serum antioxidant micronutrients and sociodemographic factors to cervical neoplasia: a case-control study. Clin Chem Lab Med. 47(8):1005-12. doi: 10.1515/CCLM.2009.221.

41.	Tomita LY, Longatto Filho A, Costa MC, et al. 2010. Diet and serum micronutrients in relation to cervical neoplasia and cancer among low-income Brazilian women. Int J Cancer. 126(3):703-14. doi: 10.1002/ijc.24793.

42.	Piyathilake CJ, Badiga S, Kabagambe EK, et al. 2012. A dietary pattern associated with LINE-1 methylation alters the risk of developing cervical intraepithelial neoplasia. Cancer Prev Res. 5(3):385-92. doi: 10.1158/1940-6207.CAPR-11-0387. Epub 2012 Jan.

43.	Ravel J, Gajer P, Abdo Z, et al. 2011. Vaginal microbiome of reproductive-age women. Proc Natl Acad Sci USA Suppl 1:4680-4687.

44.	Schellenberg JJ, Links MG, Hill JE, et al. 2011. Molecular definition of vaginal microbiota in East African commercial sex workers. Appl Environ Microbiol. 77:4066-4074.

45.	Yoshimura K, Morotomi N, Fukuda K, et al. 2011. Intravaginal microbial flora by the 16S rRNA gene sequencing. Am J Obstet Gynecol. 205:235.el-doi:10.1016/j.ajog.2011.04.018.

46.   Smith BC, McAndrew T, Chen Z, Harari A, et al. 2012. The cervical microbiome over 7 years and a comparison of methodologies for its characterization. PLoS One 7:e40425.doi:10.1371/journal.pone.0040425.

47.   Srinivasan S, Hoffman NG, Morgan MT, et al. 2012. Bacterial communities in women with bacterial vaginosis: high resolution phylogenetic analyses reveal relationships of microbiota to clinical criteria. PLoS One 7:e37818.doi:10.1371/journal.pone.0037818.

48.   Dols JAM, Reid G, Kort R, et al. 2011. PCR-based identification of eight Lactobacillus species and 18 hr-HPV genotypes in fixed cervical samples of South African women at risk of HPV and BV. Diagn Cytopathol. 40:472-477.

49.   Lee JE, Lee S, Lee H, Song YM, et al. 2013. Association of the vaginal microbiota with human papillomavirus infection in a Korean twin cohort. PLoS One. 8:63514.doi:10.1371/journal.pone.0063514.

50.   Gao W, Weng J, Gao Y, Chen X. 2013. Comparison of the vaginal microbiota diversity of women with and without human papillomavirus infection: a cross-sectional study. BMC Infect Dis. 13:271.doi:10.1186/1471-2334-13-271.

51.   Persson R, Hitti J, Verhelst R, et al. 2009. The vaginal microflora in relation to gingivitis. BMC Infect Dis. 9:6.doi:10.1186/1471-2334-9-6.

52.   Bae JH, Kim CJ, Park TC, et al. 2007. Persistence of human papillomavirus as a predictor for treatment failure after loop electrosurgical excision procedure. Int J Gynecol Cancer. 17:1271-1277.

53.   Kim YT, Lee JM, Hur SY, Cho CH, et al. 2010. Clearance of human papillomavirus infection after successful conization in patients with cervical intraepithelial neoplasia. Int J Cancer. 126:1903-1908.

54.   Jeong NH, Lee NW, Kim HJ, Kim T, Lee KW. 2009. High-risk human papillomavirus testing for monitoring patients treated for high-grade cervical intraepithelial neoplasia. J Obstet Gynaecol Res. 35:706-711.

55.   Alonso I, Torne A, Puig-Tintore LM, Esteve R, et al. 2006. Pre- and post-conization high-risk HPV testing predicts residual/recurrent disease in patients treated for CIN 2-3. Gynecol Oncol. 103:631-636.

56.   Kyrgiou M, Mitra A, Arbyn M, Stasinou S. 2014. Fertility and early pregnancy outcomes after treatment for cervical intraepithelial neoplasia: systemic review and meta-analysis. BMJ. 349:g6192.

57.   Sepkovic DW, Stein J, Carlisle AD, et al. 2009. Diindolylmethane inhibits cervical dysplasia, alters estrogen metabolism and enhances immune response in the K14-HPV16 transgenic mouse model. Cancer Epidemiol Biomarkers Prev. 18(11):2957-2964. doi: 10.1158/1055-9965.EPI-09-0698.

58.   Sepkovic DW, Raucci L, Stein J, Carlisle AD, et al. 2012. 3,3-diindolylmethane increases serum interferon-γ levels in the K14-HPV16 transgenic mouse model for cervical cancer. In Vivo. 26(12):207-11.

59.   Lenzi M, Fimognari C, Hrelia P. 2014. Sulforaphane as a promising molecule for fighting cancer. Cancer Treat Res. 159:207-23. doi: 10.1007/978-3-642-38007-5-12.

60.   Maher DM, Bell MC, O'Donnell EA, et al. 2010. Curcumin suppresses human papillomavirus oncoproteins, restores p53, Rb, and PTPN13 proteins and inhibits benzo[a]pyrene-induced upregulation of HPV E7. Molecular Carcinogenesis. 50:47-57.

61.   Singh M, Singh N. 2009. Molecular mechanism of curcumin induced cytotoxicity in human cervical carcinoma cells. Mol Cell Biochem. 325:107-119. doi: 10.1007/s11010-009-0025-5.

62.   Singh M, Singh N. 2011. Curcumin counteracts the proliferative effect of estradiol and induces apoptosis in cervical cancer cells. Mol Cell Biochem. 347(1-2):1-11. doi: 10.1007/s111010-010-06063. Epub 2010 Oct 13.

63.   Singh AK, Misra K. 2013. Human papillomavirus 16 E6 protein as a target for curcuminoids, curcumin conjugates and congeners for chemoprevention of oral and cervical cancers. Interdiscip Sci. 5(2):112-8. doi: 10.1007/s12539-013-0159-8. Epub 2013 Jun 6.

64.   Goel A, Aggarwal BB. 2010. Curcumin, the golden spice from Indian saffron, is a chemosensitizer and radiosensitizer for tumors and chemoprotector and radioprotector for normal organs. Nutrition and Cancer. 62(7):919-930. doi: 10.1080/01635581. 2010.509835.

65.   Qiao Y, Cao J, Xie L, Shi X. 2009. Cell growth inhibition and gene expression regulation by (-)-epigallocatechin-3-gallate in human cervical cancer cells. Arch Pharm Res. 32(9):1309-15. doi: 10.1007/s122272-009-1917-3. Epub 2009 Sep 26.

66.   Muthusam S, Prabakaran DS, An Z, Yu JR, Park WY. 2013. EGCG suppresses fused toes homolog protein through p53 in cervical cancer cells. Mol Biol Rep. 40(10):5587-96. doi: 10.1007/s11033-013-2660-x. Epub 2013 Sep 25.

67.   Ahn WS, Yoo J, Huh SWE, Kim CK, et al. 2003. Protective effects of green tea extracts (polyphenon E and EGCG) on human cervical lesions. Eur J Cancer Prev. 12(5):383-90.

68.   Garcia FA, Cornelison T, Nuno T, Greenspan DL, et al. 2014. Results of a phase II randomized, double-blind, placebo-controlled trial of Polyphenon E in women with persistent high-risk HPV infection and low-grade cervical intraepithelial neoplasia. Gynecol Oncol. 132(2):377-82. doi: 10.1016/j.ygyno.2013.12.034. Epub 2014 Jan 2.

69.   Oi N, Yuan J, Malakhova M, Luo K, et al. 2014. Resveratrol induces apoptosis by directly targeting Ras-GTPase-activating protein

SH3 domain-binding protein 1. Oncogene. Jul 7. doi: 10.1038/onc.2014.194.

70.   Khandayuthapani S, Marimuthu P, Hormann V, et al. 2013. Induction of apoptosis in HeLa cells via caspase activation by resveratrol and genistein. J Med Food. 16(2):139-46. doi: 10.1089/jmf.2012.0141. Epub 2013 Jan 28.

71.   Tang X, Zhang Q, Nishitani J, Brown J, Shi S, Le AD. 2007. Overexpression of human papillomavirus type 16 oncoproteins enhances hypoxia-inducible factor 1 alpha protein accumulation and vascular endothelial growth factor expression in human cervical carcinoma cells. Clin Cancer Res. 13(9):2568-76.

72.   Priyadarsini VR, Murugan SR, Maitreyi S, et al. 2010. The flavonoid quercetin induces cell cycle arrest and mitochondria-mediated apoptosis in human cervical cancer (HeLa) cells through p53 induction and NF-κB inhibition. Eur J Pharmacol. 649(1-3):84-91. doi: 10.1016/j.ejphar.2010.09.020. Epub 2010 Sep 19.

73.   Bishayee K, Ghosh S, Mukherjee A, et al. 2013. Quercetin induces cytochrome-c release and ROS accumulation to promote apoptosis and arrest the cell cycle in G2/M, in cervical carcinoma signal cascade and drug-DNA interaction. Cell Prolif. 46(2):153-63. doi: 10.1111/cpr.12017.

74.   Zhang WT, Zhang W, Zhong YJ, Lu QY, Cheng J. 2013. [Impact of quercetin on the expression of heparanase in cervical cancer cells]. Zhonhua Fu Chan Ke Za Zhi. 48(3):198-203.

75.   Macias-Barragan J, Caligiuri A, Garcia-Banuelos J, et al. 2014. [Effects of alpha lipoic acid and pirfenidone on liver cells antioxidant modulation against oxidative damage]. Rev Med Chil. 142(12):1553-64. doi: 10.4067/S0034-98872014001200009.

76.   Lee SG, Lee CG, Yun DY, Yang JW, Kim HW. 2012. Effect of lipoic acid on expression of angiogenic factors in diabetic rat retina. Clin Experiment Ophthalmol. 40(1):e47-57. doi: 10.1111/j.1442-9071.2011.02695.x. Epub 2011 Nov 4.

77.   Yoo TH, Lee JH, Chun HS, Chi SG. 2013. α-lipoic acid prevents p53 degradation in colon cancer cells by blocking NF-κB induction of RPS6KA4. Anticancer Drugs. 24(6):555-65. doi: 10.1097/CAD.0b013e32836181eb.

78.   Gorelick C, Lopez-Jones M, Goldberg GL, Romney SL, Khabele D. 2004. Coenzyme Q10 and lipid-related gene induction in HeLa cells. Am J Obstet Gynecol. 190(5):1432-4.

79.   Gutierrez-Mariscal FM, Perez-Martinez P, Delgado-Lista J, et al. 2012. Mediterranean diet supplemented with coenzyme Q10 induces postprandial changes in p53 in response to oxidative DNA damage in elderly subjects. Age. 34(2):389-403.doi: 10.1007/s11357-011-9229-1. Epub 2011 Mar 15.

80.   Choi JS, Park SY, Yi EY, Kim YJ, Jeong JW. 2011. Coenzyme Q10 decreases basic fibroblast growth factor (bFGF)-induced angiogenesis by blocking ERK activation. Oncol Res. 19(10-11):455-61.

81.   Jing L, He MT, Chang Y, Mehta SL, He QP, Zhang JZ, Li PA. 2015. Coenzyme Q10 protects astrocytes from ROS-induced damage though inhibition of mitochondria-mediated cell death pathway. Int J Biol Sci. 11(1):59-66. doi: 10.7150/ijbs.10174. eCollection 2015.

82.   Acharya A, Das I, Singh S, Saha T. 2010. Chemopreventive properties of indole-3-carbinol, diindolylmethane and other constituents of cardamom against carcinogenesis. Recent Patents on Food, Nutrition and Agriculture. 2:166-77.

83.   Kandaola PK, Srivastava SK. 2012. DIMming ovarian cancer growth. Curr Drug Targets. 13(14):1869-75.

84.   Malhotra A, Nair P, Dhawan DK. 2014. Study to evaluate molecular mechanics behind synergistic chemo-preventive effects of curcumin and resveratrol during lung carcinogenesis. PLoS One, 9(4):1-9. E93820.

85.   Peng S, Trimble C, Wu L, Pardoll D, et al. 2007. HLA-DQB1*02-restricted HPV-16 E7 peptide-specific CD4+ T-cell immune responses correlate with regression of HPV-16-associated high-grade squamous intraepithelial lesions. Clin Cancer Res. 13(8):2479-2487. doi: 10.1158/1078-0432.CCR-06-2916.

86.   Scardamaglia P, Carraro C, Mancino P, Stentella P. 2010. [Effectiveness of the treatment with beta-glucan in the HPV-CIN 1 lesions]. Minerva Ginecol. 62(5):389-93.

87.   Vetvicka V, Vetvickova J. 2014. Immune-enhancing effects of Maitake (Grifola frondosa) and Shiitake (Lentinula edodes) extracts. Ann Transl Med. 2(2):14. doi: 10.3978/j.issn.2305-5839.2014.01.05.

88.   Sorice A, Guerriero E, Capone F, Colonna G, et al. 2014. Ascorbic acid: Its role in immune system and chronic inflammation diseases. Mini Rev Med Chem. 14(5):444-52.

89.   Li X, Qu L, Dong Y, Han L, Liu E, et al. 2014. A review of recent research progress on the astragalus genus. Molecules. 19(11):18850-18880.

90.   Munagala R, Kausar H, Munjal C, Gupta RC. 2011. Withaferin A induces p53-dependent apoptosis by repression of HPV oncogenes and upregulation of tumor suppressor proteins in human cervical cancer cells. Carcinogenesis. 32(11):1697-705. doi: 10.1093/carcin/bgr192. Epub 2011 Aug 22.

91.   Mishra LC, Singh BB, Dagenais S. 2000. Scientific basis for the therapeutic use of Withania somnifera (ashwagandha): a review. Altern Med Rev. 5(4):334-46.

92.   Vetvicka V, Vetvickova J. 2011. Immune enhancing effects of WB365, a novel combination of ashwagandha (Withania somnifera) and

maitake (Grifola frondosa) extracts. N Am J Med Sci. 3(7):320-24. doi: 10.4297/najms.2011.3320.

93.   Hwang JH, Kim MK, Lee JK. 2010. Dietary supplements reduce the risk of cervical intraepithelial neoplasia. Int J Gynecol. 20(3):398-403. doi: 10.1111/IGC.0b013e318d02ff2.

94.   Verhoeven V, Renard N, Makar A, Van Royen P, et al. 2013. Probiotics enhance the clearance of human papillomavirus-related cervical lesions: a prospective controlled pilot study. Eur J Cancer Prev. 22(1):46-51. doi: 10.1097/CEJ.0b013e328355ed23.

95.   Cha MK, Lee DK, An HM, Lee SW, et al. 2012. Antiviral activity of Bifidobacterium adolescentis SPM1005-A on human papillomavirus type 16. BMC Med. 10:72. doi: 10.1186/1741-7015-10-72.

96.   Schulte-Uebbing C, Schlett S, Craiut I, Antal L, Olah H. 2014. Chronic cervical infections and dysplasia (CIN 1, CIN 2): vaginal vitamin D (high doses) treatment: a new effective method? Dermatoendocrinol. 6(1):e27791. doi: 10.4161/derm.27791. Epub 2014 Jan 20.

97.   Shen SS, Hamamoto ST, Bern HA, Steinhardt RA. 1978. Alteration of sodium transport in mouse mammary epithelium associated with neoplastic transformation. Cancer Res. 38:1356-1361.

98.   Kaplan JG. 1978. Membrane cation transport and the control of proliferation of mammalian cells. Ann Rev Physiol. 40:19-41.

99.   Kimelberg H, Kimelberg E. 1975. Increased ouabain-sensitive 86Rb+ uptake and sodium and potassium ion-activated adenosine triphosphatase activity in transformed cell lines. J Biol Chem. 250:100-104.

100.   Alevizopoulos K, Calogeropoulou T, Lang F, Stournaras C. 2014. Na+/K+ ATPase inhibitors in cancer. Curr Drug Targets. 15(10): 988-1000.

101.   Lefranc F, Kiss R. 2008. The sodium pump alpha 1 subunit as a potential target to combat apoptosis-resistant glioblastomas. Neoplasia. 10(3):198-206.

102.   McConkey DJ, Lin Y, Nutt LK, Ozel HZ, Newman RA. 2000. Cardiac glycosides stimulate Ca2+ increases and apoptosis in androgen-independent, metastatic human prostate adenocarcinoma cells. Cancer Res. 60(14):3807-3812.

103.   Huang YT, Chueh SC, Teng CM, Guh JH. 2004. Investigation of ouabain-induced anticancer effect in human androgen-independent prostate cancer PC-3 cells. Biochem Pharmacol. 67(4):727-733.

104.   Mijatovic T, Roland I, Van Quaquebeke E, Nilsson B, Mathieu. 2007. The alpha-1 subunit of the sodium pump could represent a novel target to combat non-small cell lung cancers. J Pathol. 212(2):170—179.

105.   Mijatovic T, Op De Beeck A, Van Quaquebeke E, Dewelle J, et al. 2006. The cardenolide UNBS1450 is able to deactivate nuclear factor

kappaB-mediated cytoprotective effects in human non-small cell lung cancer cells. Mol Cancer Ther. 5(2):391-399.

106.   Stenkvist B. 2001. Cardenolides and cancer. Anti-Cancer Drugs. 12(7):635-638.

107.   Janovska M, Kubala M, Simanek V, Ulrichova J. 2010. Interaction of sanguinarine and its dihydroderivative with the Na+/K+-ATPase. Complex view on the old problem. Toxicol Lett. 196(1):56-9. doi: 10.1016/j.toxlet.2010.03.1114. Epub 2010 Apr 10.

108.   Xu JY, Meng QH, Chong Y, Jiao Y, et al. 2012. Sanguinarine inhibits growth of human cervical cancer cells through the induction of apoptosis. Oncol Rep. 28(6):2264-70. doi: 10.3892/or.2012.2024. Epub 2012 Sep 11.

109.   Scheiner-Bobis G. 2001. Sanguinarine induces K+ outflow from yeast cells expressing mammalian sodium pumps. Naunyn Schmiedebergs Arch Pharmacol. 363(2):203-8.

110.   Weidmann H. 2005. Na/K-ATPase, endogenous digitalis like compounds and cancer development—a hypothesis. Front Biosci. 10:2165-2176.

111.   Mijatovic T, Ingrassia L, Facchini V, Kiss R. 2008. Na+/K+-ATPase alpha subunits as new targets in anticancer therapy. Expert Opin Ther Targets. 12(11):1403-1417.

112.   Xu ZW, Wang FM, Gao MJ, Chen XY, Hu WL, Xu RC. 2010. Targeting the Na+/K+-ATPase alpha1 subunit of hepatoma HepG2 cell line to induce apoptosis and cell cycle arresting. Biol Pharm Bull. 33(5):743-751.

113.   Prassas I, Diamandis EP. 2008. Novel therapeutic applications of cardiac glycosides. Nat Rev Drug Discov. 7(11):926-935.

114.   Mirzaie-Kashani E, Bouzari M, Talebi A, Arbabzadeh-Zavareh F. 2014. Detection of human papillomavirus in chronic cervicitis, cervical adenocarcinoma, intraepithelial neoplasia and squamous cell carcinoma. Jundishapur J Microbiol. 7(5):e990. doi: 10.5812/jjm.9930. Epub 2014 May 1.

115.   Basu P, Dutta S, Begum R, Mittal S, Dutta PD, et al. 2013. Clearance of cervical human papillomavirus infection by topical application of curcumin and curcumin containing polyherbal cream: a phase II randomized controlled study. Asian Pac J Cancer Prev. 14(10):5753-9.

116.   Debata PR, Castellanos MR, Fata JE, Baggett S, et al. 2012. A novel curcumin-based vaginal cream Vacurin selectively eliminates apposed human cervical cancer cells. Gynecol Oncol. 129(1):145-53. doi: 10.1016/j.ygyno.2012.12.005. Epub 2012 Dec 9.

117.   Talwar GP, Dar SA, Rai MK, Reddy KV, et al. 2008. A novel polyherbal microbicide with inhibitory effect on bacterial, fungal and

viral genital pathogens. Int J Antimicrob Agents. 32(2):180-5. doi: 10.1016/j.ijantimicag.2008..03.004. Epub 2008 Jun20.

118.   van de Wijgert JH, Borgdorff H, Verheist R, et al. 2014. The vaginal microbiota: What have we learned after a decade of molecular characterization? PLoS One. 9(8): e105998. doi: 10.1371/journal.pone.0105998.

119.   Schulte-Uebbing C, Schlett S, Craiut I, Antal L, Olah H. 2014. Chronic cervical infections and dysplasia (CIN1, CIN2): vaginal vitamin D (high dose) treatment: A new effective method? Dermatoendocrinol. 6(1): e27791. doi: 10.4161/derm.27791. Epub 2014 Jan 20.

Appendix A: Discharge of Patient

Abandoned

by Dr. Nick LeRoy

For many of us, the relationship with our doctor is based upon trust and respect. In fact, the degree to which we value our doctor is directly proportionate to our trust in his or her opinion and perceived wisdom that accompanies this opinion. It is with the hope of wisdom and sound advice that we seek medical care in general.

This relationship with a physician is significant because it is difficult, if not impossible, to navigate a health condition without advanced training in anatomy, physiology, biochemistry, pathology, laboratory diagnostics and many, many other areas of advanced study. Thus, we are dependent upon others (physicians) to assist us in determining the state of disease and available treatments when necessary. **This dependency makes us particularly vulnerable, especially in our greatest time of need when confronted with a life-threatening disease.**

But what happens when this physician in whom we place great trust; in whose knowledge, opinion and advice we seek; doesn't trust and respect *you*? Or more specifically, how do you respond when your doctor fails to appreciate fully the invested interest that you have in your own body and the right that we all maintain in that regard?

The document that follows this article is the correspondence sent via certified mail to a patient whom I treated for a persistently high-grade pap lesion that was consistently negative on biopsy. As you can see, the letter states that her gynecologist would no longer be her doctor because the patient did not follow her advice. Her doctor was insistent that she have part of her cervix removed surgically, and rather than undergo this invasive procedure, she first chose to try the alternative treatment that I provide.

Now perhaps I am naïve, but I maintain that what a person does with his or her own body is his or her own decision. The ideal scenario in deciding how to treat an illness always consists of getting more than one opinion, educating oneself regarding the disease in question, and then acting in a way that we believe is in our best interest. I actually do something similar with my car: I take it to my mechanic, get his opinion, and if I don't like it, I go get another opinion. But when I go back to my original mechanic, he certainly doesn't refuse to work on my car because I didn't follow his initial advice.

What happened to this patient is abandonment, pure and simple. It is fundamentally an egoic, my-way-or-the-highway bullying of a woman who is scared and in need. It is devoid of compassion. It is arrogant. **It represents much of what is lacking in medicine**

and the antithesis of what we seek in a doctor. This woman was not abandoning her doctor in seeking alternative care, but was only using another "mechanic" with a different perspective. It was the patient's intent, in fact, to continue care with this doctor and clinic after undergoing the escharotic treatments that I provided for her.

 I say all of this knowing full well why this women's clinic discharged her as a patient: she was viewed as a risk; in other words, her doctor was afraid that if she underwent alternative treatment that didn't work, she would turn around and sue the doctor. As ridiculous as this might seem--because how can the doctor be liable when she told the patient very clearly to have surgery--this is part of the "risk management" that is taught to all medical students. It is commonplace and considered the standard in dealing with "difficult" patients. But is it moral? Is it compassionate? **Or is it instead the ego of a doctor miffed because a patient is questioning her authority?**

Earlier I posed the question "how do you respond when your doctor" abandons you. I don't know that there is a good answer, but I think it may be along these lines: the doctor in whom you trusted may not have been such a great doctor after all. Maybe you're better off without him or her. **Maybe he or she was an asshole all along and maybe you should send a certified letter back attesting to this supposition.** Or simply, good riddance (with a bad online review, of course)! I think that this last recommendation is best: let prospective patients of the doctor know that he or she expects patients to step-in-line, don't ask too many questions, and to do as told.

Incidentally, I treated this woman ten times with an escharotic applied to her cervix and all of her pap tests have been normal ever since. Additionally, the virus (HR-HPV) that was the cause of the pre-cancer was eliminated.

Obstetrics and Gynecology

BUSINESS CENTER

Director

OFFICE LOCATIONS

March 22, 2013

Dear

Dr. ░░░ had recommended a leep procedure as a result of the pathology from your Colposcopy February, 12, 2013. The result of high grade squamous cells was noted and discussed with you. Abnormalities or changes noted can indicate precancer or cancer. The procedure ordered for you can determine the difference between continued health and the need for immediate care. You have not scheduled your leep procedure as of today.

I am writing to you to advise you that ░░░ will no longer be able to provide you your gynecological care beginning April 22, 2013. This letter will serve as notification that you have 30 days to find a new gynecologist. Should a medical emergency arise during this time, we will treat you according to medical legal guidelines.

If you have chosen to seek medical care elsewhere regarding your leep procedure, please notify our office. I have enclosed a medical release form for you to fill out and return to our office. Upon receipt, we will then forward your records to your physician.

Sincerely,

Office Administrator

Certified & Regular Mail

Appendix B: Recipes

Eggs with Greens

- 1-2 eggs
- 1 ½ cups of "Dr. Nick's Veggie Mix" or arugula, collard greens or kale
- 1 tsp. coconut oil
- Salt/pepper

Put oil in a heated skillet and add the greens. Crack the egg(s) over the greens. Season with salt and pepper. Cover skillet and cook on low heat for about 7 minutes or until yolks are cooked.

Additional vegetables can be added if desired. I'm lazy, so I don't stir in the eggs; I just cover and walk away for a few minutes.

Green Smoothie

- 1 cup of "Dr. Nick's Veggie Mix" or other greens/cabbage
- ¼ carrot
- ¼ beet
- ¼ package of silken tofu (a vegan or rice protein powder can be used for more protein)
- ¼ apple or 1/8 cup of frozen berries (or both)
- 1 cup of water

Put all ingredients in juice extractor container. Blend for twenty seconds.

This recipe can be varied but the goal is to have more greens than carrot, beet and fruits which are all high in sugar. Sometimes I add ginger root or garlic clove—both of which are great for the immune system.

Greens and Beans

- 1 cup mixed beans (pre-cooked)
- 1 cup "Dr. Nick's Veggie Mix" or other greens
- 1 tbs coconut oil or olive oil
- 1 tsp. Walker's Woods™ Jamaican Jerk Paste or Patak's™ curry paste or other seasoning

Put oil in a skillet and add beans and seasoning then stir. Add greens. Let simmer for a few minutes until the greens are wilted. Water should be added if too dry.

I like to cook my own beans rather than use canned beans which will have a plastic lining that is toxic. I purchase about 1.5 cups each of a whole bunch of different dried beans (mung, adzuki, white, navy, black, garbanzo, lentil, etc.) and mix them together. When I want to make beans I soak them overnight, drain, add water and cook on low heat for about 2 hours. I always make enough for several meals.

Acknowledgments

Thanks to all of my patients who entrusted me with your health. Without your support I would not be in practice and this book would not exist.

Thank you Mitch Hagan for providing the cover design of this book. Mitch is my talented graphic design/marketing expert to which I defer in all things relating to print media.

Thank you Jeanne Farnan, MD for editing my book. Your suggestions helped to make it better. Dr. Farnan is an associate professor of internal medicine at the University of Chicago Medicine.

Thank you Frank Yurasek, Ph. D. for being a mentor and partner in our first clinic. It was your penchant for creativity, bees and other eccentric therapies that helped set me on this path.

A special thanks to my friends and family and to Tamar, who has endured my difficult nature with a heart like no other.

Most of all, thank you LeeAnn and Roger for always being supportive and overall amazing parents.

Nicholas LeRoy, DC, MS

Dr. Nick LeRoy is a holistic physician who integrates his training in nutrition, chiropractic, acupuncture, internal medicine and women's health to offer unique approaches for most ailments. Dr. LeRoy was a primary care physician for Alternative Medicine Incorporated, a Blue Cross Blue Shield HMO. He is also a member of the American Academy of Chiropractic Physicians.

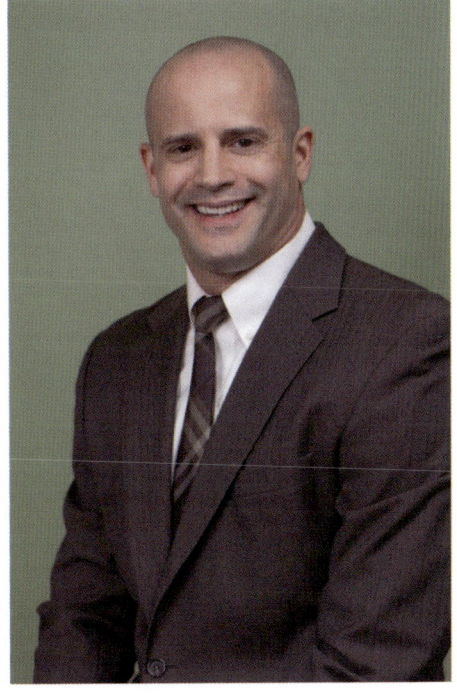

Dr. LeRoy has been featured as a women's health expert at the Whole Life Expo of 1996, 1997, 1998 and 2002, and he has been featured on Chicago NBC news, ABC news, Fox news and local radio as a holistic medicine expert. He has also lectured on breast cancer prevention and treatment at Gilda's Club of Chicago and the Wellness House in Hinsdale, IL.

Dr. LeRoy holds a BS in human biology from the University of Wisconsin at Milwaukee, where he also completed post-graduate studies in molecular biology and endocrinology. He graduated summa cum laude from the National University of Health Sciences, and graduated from Midwest Center for the Study of Oriental Medicine. Dr. LeRoy has a Master's Degree in Advanced Clinical Practice as well as post-doctoral training in internal medicine and gynecology.

Dr. LeRoy has been in private practice since 1995. He was also credentialed by NCQA as a primary care physician for HMO-Illinois from 2000 to 2017. In addition to this experience, Dr. LeRoy was the past CEO of a company providing interactive corporate health and wellness programs, services and resources. He has also been on the faculty of several schools teaching anatomy, physiology and pathology.

Dr. Nick began his journey into HPV and cervical dysplasia in 1995, when he offered a unique alternative approach to treating cervical dysplasia to a patient who refused to have a LEEP for CIN2. After the successful treatment of this first patient, Dr. Nick wrote about it in his newsletter and his article was reprinted in *Holistic Chicago* magazine. And so began his twenty-five year endeavor to help women to overcome this condition.

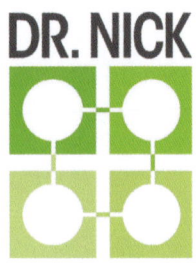

Dr. Nick is available for Skype consultations. For additional information go to his website at *drnickleroy.com.* Dr. Nick can be contacted at **312.343.6425** or *drnickfrontdesk@gmail.com.*

Printed in Great Britain
by Amazon

24480930R00071